CONTENTS

How to Use the Student Workbook for Lees' *Skin Care, Beyond the Basics*, 4th Ed.

After reading each chapter, this workbook is designed to reinforce and help cement the terminology and concepts you are introduced to in the text *Skin Care, Beyond the Basics*, 4th Ed. Because this text takes you to the next level, there may be terms you are already familiar with, though as more advanced concepts are introduced, this workbook that accompanies Lees' text will help you learn the material. Different people learn in many different ways. There are a variety of learning enforcement activities offered in this workbook, including multiple choice questions, true or false questions, fill in the blank with word banks provided of different terminology and key words, short-answer questions about important concepts, and fun puzzles that include word scrambles and word finds using key terms.

This workbook uses many different types of learning enforcement activities in which students may go back and forth between the text and the workbook to find answers if they need to—it is designed to work well with your text. Having fun puzzles is a unique way this workbook will help students understand and apply the most important concepts and services described within this workbook. The following are examples of the activities within the student workbook.

Samples of Workbook Activities

Multiple Choice Questions

1. Estheticians evaluate and apply services to promote the health of:
   a. Muscles   c. The heart
   b. Skin   d. The lungs

Here the answer would be: b. Skin

True/False Questions

_____ Estheticians help promote the health and appearance of skin.

The correct answer would be true, so place a "T" in the line provided.

Short Answer

What is OSHA?

Occupational Safety and Health Administration. A federal government agency, part of the Department of Labor, formed to help ensure that places of employment maintain a safe and healthy environment for employees.

Write the correct answer (which has been provided for you in above).

Word Scramble

Unscramble the key terms below and write the term inside the cells, by using the definitions shown.

---

iksn
skin _ _ _ _ _ _ _ _ _ _ _ _ _   a layer of epithelial tissue that covers the body

tyuabe
Beauty _ _ _ _ _ _ _ _ _ _ _   a subjective opinion on how esthetically pleasing a person or thing is

---

Using the definition provided to the left of the scrambled term, write the correctly spelled term next to its matching definition.

Word Find

skin   Beauty

Circle the terms that are related to the correlating chapter. Words may be vertical, horizontal, diagonal, or backwards.

S	F	E	R	S	R	R	U	S	B	V
W	X	Y	F	X	I	Q	R	**K**	T	X
X	X	X	U	X	L	X	X	**I**	X	P
W	R	**B**	**E**	**A**	**U**	**T**	**Y**	N	Z	A
T	E	X	G	X	A	X	T	X	S	T
W	R	X	U	X	X	X	F	Y	X	H

Purpose

We hope that this workbook will be both educational and fun as you navigate through Lees' *Skin Care: Beyond the Basics*, 4th Ed. The world of esthetics is both rewarding and fulfilling and we look forward to helping you discover more advanced concepts and skills within the wonderful world of skin care. Enjoy.

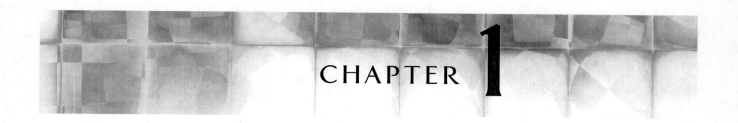

CHAPTER 1

Advanced Anatomy and Physiology of the Skin

Multiple Choice

Circle the correct answer.

1. Cells are
   A. the building blocks of the human body. Within each cell, many chemical and physical processes are taking place continually.

   B. a network of lipids and protein in the body.

   C. special structures that provide communication between tissues, organs, and different parts of the body.

   D. small structures that contain hereditary traits.

2. The name of the outer shell of a cell is the
   A. nucleus.　　　B. cell membrane.　　　C. cytoplasm.　　　D. mitochondria.

3. The cell is nourished by
   A. the receptor sites.　　B. the fluid in the cytoplasm.　　C. ribosomes.　　D. the blood.

4. The function of the cell membrane is to
   A. help break down sugars and fats.

   B. act as a storage unit for waste and excess food supplies.

   C. give the cell structure and shape.

   D. help convert oxygen to carbon dioxide in the cell for proper waste control.

5. The receptor sites are
   A. demolition crews that manufacture enzymes that break down molecules too large to enter the cells.

   B. structures inside the cells that form little canals within the cytoplasm that allow substances and other organelles to move around.

   C. located on the cell membrane and act as a communication system between cells, tissues, and different parts of the body.

   D. primarily used for the division of the cells.

6. Which is an example of how a receptor site works?
   A. It is a switch that is turned on when the male hormones stimulate the receptor sites with the production of sebum in the cells of the sebaceous gland.

   B. It provides proteins that break down simple sugars, fats, and parts of proteins so they can be used for energy by the cell.

   C. By acting as the digestive system of the cell, they convert oxygen and nutrients that can be used as energy for the cell.

   D. With its gel-like consistency, it allows other structures to move around inside the cell.

7. Cytoplasm is
   A. a storage mechanism that helps store proteins for later conversion to manufacture necessary chemicals when the cell needs them.

   C. the outer shell of the cell that gives it shape and structure and contains many of the internal parts of the cell.

   B. a gel-like fluid located in the cell made up of water and other substances that allows other structures to move around inside the cell.

   D. a miniature body organ within the cell, each with its own function.

8. Organelles are
   A. very small, self-contained units of life.

   C. the lungs and digestive system of the cell.

   B. receptor sites that receive chemical messages from other cells or organs that cause the cells to behave in a certain way.

   D. small structures within each cell, each with its own function.

9. The endoplasmic reticulum is
   A. a cell that provides communication between the different tissues, organs, and parts of the body.

   C. a process where the cell membrane can let substances into the cell, such as food, water, and oxygen, and conversely let substances out, such as waste and carbon dioxide.

   B. a maze-like structure of material that forms little canals within the cytoplasm and allows substances and organelles to move around.

   D. very small organelles that help build protein structures that the cell needs.

10. Mitochondria are
    A. the lungs and the digestive system of the cell.

    C. located in the nucleus of the cell.

    B. storage units for waste and excess food supplies.

    D. the smallest organelles.

Parts of the Cell

Identify and label the parts of the cell.

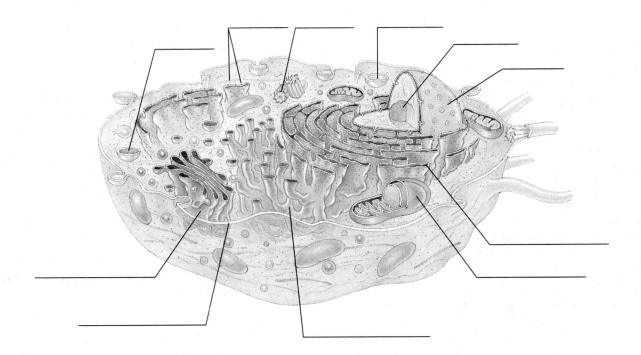

True/False

Write T for true and F for false in the space provided.

1. ____ Amino acids are proteins used by the cell for energy.

2. ____ A storage mechanism that helps store proteins for later conversion is the Golgi apparatus.

3. ____ Vacuoles are small organelles that help build protein structures the cell needs.

4. ____ Receptor sites manufacture enzymes that help break apart large molecules entering the cell so that they can be more easily converted to other necessary chemicals and substances.

5. ____ Ribosomes are one of the largest of the organelles, and they act as storage vats for waste.

6. ____ Adenosine triphosphate (ATP) can be considered as a ready-to-use energy packet that can be used by any organelle in the cell.

Fill in the Blank

Using the word bank below, fill in the blank to complete the sentence. The same word may be used more than once.

Word Bank

cytoplasm	lungs	guard	endoplasmic	hormones
cell membrane	broken down	ribosomes	reticulum	Golgi apparatus
absorbed	oxygen	vacuoles	lysosomes	kidneys
blood	mitochondria		carbon dioxide	

The _____ delivers food to the cell that has already been _____ _____ by the digestive system, _____ through the intestinal wall, and absorbed by the blood. The blood also delivers _____ from the ____. First, the cell membrane acts as a ____ allowing certain substances into the _____. Once inside, these substances may be guided to their destination by the canals of the _____ _____. The _____ start breaking down the large protein molecules. The _____ build or rebuild the proteins the cell needs at the time. The _____ serve as power plants, making usable energy for the cell from the variety of proteins, sugars, oxygen, and fats. Excess food products and waste from production are stored in the _____. The _____ _____ stores proteins to use later for manufacturing enzymes and _____. After production is over, waste materials and _____ _____ are released by the ___ _____ into the blood. The _____ takes the waste away to the ____, where the _____ _____ is expelled, and to the _____, which filter out the other waste.

Matching

Match the term with the best description, and write the letter of the term in the space provided.

Description   *Terms*

1. ____ Brain of the cell.   A. mitosis

2. ____ Duplicates itself and gives directions for cell operations.   B. genes

3. ____ The process by which cells divide.   C. nucleus

4. ____ The small structures responsible for hereditary traits.   D. DNA

5. ____ New structures begin migrating to the opposite ends of the cell during   E. swelling
        this time.

6. ____ Group of cells that perform the same function.   F. third phase

7. ____ Blood is mostly made of this substance.   G. red blood cells

8. ____ Completes transport of oxygen and carbon dioxide to and from the cells.   H. white corpuscles

9. ____ Liquid that helps filter waste from the bloodstream.   I. lymph nodes

10. ____ Body system filters located in armpits, groin, and neck.   J. plasma

11. ____ Responsible for defending the body against bacterial invasion.   K. lymph

12. ____ This condition can arise when the lymph nodes are filtering out bacteria   L. tissues and debris.

Matching

Match the term with the best description, and write the letter of the term in the space provided.

Description   *Terms*

1. ____ Responsible for involuntary muscle actions.   A. connective tissue

2. ____ Responsible for the movement of the bones.   B. epithelial tissue

3. ____ Classified in a separate category as both striated and involuntary.   C. nerve tissue

4. ____ Cartilage and ligaments are examples of this type of tissue that connects   D. liquid tissue
        bones to bones and bones to muscle.

5. ____ Makes up the bones of the body.   E. skeletal tissue

6. ____ Controls the brain and the nerves.   F. adipose tissue

7. ____ Includes blood and lymph and is responsible for carrying oxygen   G. endothelial tissue
        and blood to all cells.

8. ____ Fat tissue.   H. cardiac tissue

9. ____ Refers to tissue that lines the outer and exposed body surfaces.   I. visceral tissue

10. ____ Refers to tissue that lines the walls of the intestines, lungs,   J. skeletal muscle tissue
        and other organs.

True/False

Write T for true and F for false in the space provided.

1. ____ The subcutaneous layer is the most internal layer of skin that provides cushioning.

2. ____ The second layer of the skin, the dermis, is often called the "dead" layer.

3. ____ The stratum granulosum is called the "live" layer.

4. ____ The stratum corneum is also called the "horny" layer.

5. ____ The epidermis is the outermost layer of the three basic layers of the skin.

6. ____ The stratum lucidum is the layer of the skin that has little spines on the outside of the cell membranes.

7. ____ The innermost layer of the epidermis is the basal layer.

8. ____ The stratum granulosum, located in the epidermis, is filled with keratohyalin, which helps to form keratin.

Multiple Choice

Circle the correct answer.

1. Lamellated corpuscles are nerve endings found in which layer of the skin?
   A. subcutaneous layer   B. dermis layer   C. epidermis layer   D. basal layer

2. Which sublayer is found at the base of the dermis of the skin?
   A. papillary layer   B. subcutaneous layer   C. stratum spinosum layer   D. reticular layer

3. Which sublayer is found in the upper portion of the dermis?
   A. reticular layer   B. stratum granulosum   C. papillary layer   D. stratum corneum

4. Where are the Meissner's corpuscles found?
   A. basal layer   B. reticular layer of   C. papillary layer of   D. subcutaneous layer
                              the dermis   the dermis

5. This layer contains nerve endings called lamellated corpuscles, which are responsive to pressure.
   A. epidermis   B. dermis   C. stratum corneum   D. subcutaneous layer

6. Which layer contains collagen and elastin fibrils?
   A. epidermis   B. reticular layer of the   C. papillary of the dermis   D. subcutaneous layer
                              dermis

7. This substance is flexible and gives the skin its ability to "bounce back."
   A. collagen   B. papillary layer   C. reticular layer   D. elastin

8. This substance is not flexible and gives the skin its firmness and inability to stretch.
   A. collagen   B. papillary layer   C. reticular layer   D. elastin

9. There are approximately how many types of collagen?
   A. 16   B. 3   C. 25   D. 8

10. Collagen is manufactured by these types of cells.
    A. epithelial   B. fibroblasts   C. adenosine triphosphate   D. amino acid

11. Which gland is responsible for the production of sebum?
    A. sudoriferous   B. sebaceous   C. eccrine   D. apocrine

12. What is the substance between the cells in the epidermis?
    A. lymph   B. sebum   C. sweat   D. interstitial fluid

Fill in the Blank

Using the word bank below, fill in the blank to complete the sentence. The same word may be used more than once.

Word Bank

transepidermal water
  loss (TEWL)
protein keratin
  synthesis
stratum corneum

melanocytes
hormones
granular
eccrine glands

sweat
stratum spinosum
stratum lucidum
fats

lamellar bodies
eleidin
apocrine
melanin

stratum granulosum
corneocytes
lipids
keratin

1. The interstitial fluid prevents _____ _____ _____.

2. The sudoriferous glands produce _____.

3. The _____ glands are present in the groin and armpits and produce body odor.

4. The sweat glands present on the face are called _____ _____.

5. _____ is a mixture of water, salt, urea, uric acid, and ammonia.

6. Pigment-producing _____ are found in the basal layer of the epidermis.

7. Pigment found in the skin is called _____.

8. Melanin production can be stimulated by _____.

9. As a type of protein, _____ can protect the skin against invasion by certain substances.

10. _____ help to hold the keratinized cells together.

11. The process of _____ _____ _____ begins in the basal layer, where fibrils begin to form from the cytoplasm in the cell.

12. The _____ _____ layer is so named because the cells appear to have little spines on the outside of the cell membranes.

13. The _____ _____ layer is so named because the cells are filled with a substance called keratohyalin, which helps form keratin. The cells in this layer begin to look granular.

14. In the _____ stage, lipids are formed to help serve as a medium or mortar for the outer cell layer.

15. The _____ _____ is the clear layer of the skin.

16. _____ is a substance produced from keratohyalin that eventually forms keratin.

17. The outermost or "horny" layer of the skin is the _____ _____.

18. Cells in the stratum corneum layer are referred to as _____.

19. _____ _____ produce more lipids, which permits certain substances in and out of the "mortar" of the cell layer.

20. The ___ formed by the lamellar bodies serve almost the same purpose as the cell membrane by allowing certain substances in and gases and toxins out of the skin.

Short Answer

1. Drugs can penetrate the skin _____ .

2. Name four ways that substances can penetrate the skin.

   A. _____

   B. _____

C. _____

D. _____

3. Name the order of permeability of various areas of the body.

A. _____

B. _____

C. _____

D. _____

E. _____

4. What area of the face is more penetrable and why?

_____

_____

5. Name two factors concerning the skin that can influence penetration potential.

A. _____

B. _____

6. If skin is injured, it is said to have what, and what does it mean?

_____

_____

7. By what can the barrier function be injured?

_____

_____

_____

8. What is it about a substance or product that can affect permeability?

_____

9. Name four ingredients that have small molecular structures and more affinity for lipids.

A. _____

B. _____

C. _____

D. _____

10. Name an ingredient that does not penetrate.

_____

11. Name three products that should not be allowed to penetrate the skin.

A. _____

B. _____

C. _____

12. Why is the thickness of the stratum corneum a factor in permeability?

_____

_____

13. What is there about oily skin that affects penetration?

   _____

   _____

14. How does the temperature of the skin affect penetration?

   _____

   _____

15. When dealing with excessively oily skin, how do you prepare it to make it more permeable?

   _____

   _____

16. Name four ways to remove excess corneocytes from the skin.

   A. _____

   B. _____

   C. _____

   D. _____

17. Name four ways the skin is improved by removing dead skin cells.

   A. _____

   B. _____

   C. _____

   D. _____

18. Name four ways to exfoliate the skin.

   A. _____

   B. _____

   C. _____

   D. _____

19. Name two (nonequipment) techniques that you as an esthetician can use to affect permeability.

   A. _____

   B. _____

20. How does massage affect permeability?

   _____

   _____

   _____

21. Give examples of heat and cold treatments that can affect permeability.

   Heat treatments: _____

   Cold treatments: _____

22. How does the selection of treatment cream affect permeability?

   _____

   _____

   _____

   _____

23. Name two types of equipment that increase the penetration ability of a product into the skin.

_____

_____

_____

24. Why is wet skin more receptive to penetration than dry skin?

_____

_____

_____

25. What is occlusion?

_____

_____

_____

Define

Use the space provided to define these terms.

1. Basal layer

2. Fibroblasts

3. Ground substance

4. Glycosaminoglycans (GAGs)

5. Stratum corneum

6. Stratum spinosum

7. Stratum granulosum

_____

_____

_____

8. Stratum lucidum

_____

_____

_____

9. Hyaluronic acid

_____

_____

_____

10. Desquamation

_____

_____

_____

Word Search

Find the following terms in the word search. Find the 15 terms that are related to or are structures of the skin:

sweat	melanocytes	lipids	collagen
apocrine	melanin	protein	granulosum
eccrine	hormones	stratum	elastin
glands	keratin	spinosum	

```
C  D  G  K  S  M  O  A  P  O  C  R  I  N  E
M  P  T  A  T  O  P  Z  R  Q  R  U  Y  A  L
S  K  G  P  R  S  T  H  O  R  M  O  N  E  S
W  U  R  X  A  E  K  J  T  L  E  E  W  Q  P
E  L  A  S  T  I  N  E  E  W  L  U  Q  A  I
A  L  N  L  U  X  D  P  I  J  A  T  U  R  N
T  Y  U  K  M  E  L  A  N  I  N  R  Y  E  O
N  E  L  W  T  X  T  D  S  F  O  L  G  Y  S
T  C  O  L  L  A  G  E  N  L  C  L  L  K  U
G  C  S  Q  A  W  R  X  U  T  Y  D  A  P  M
V  R  U  T  L  L  K  E  R  A  T  I  N  O  O
A  I  M  C  L  L  L  L  C  L  E  L  D  O  P
Z  N  H  L  F  L  I  P  I  D  S  L  S  J  H
Z  E  H  L  F  P  K  L  M  Q  S  L  S  J  H
```

Word Scramble

Unscramble the key terms below and write the term inside the cells, by using the definitions shown.

ealinnm

- - - - - - - - - - - - - - - - -   the substance that produces our skin's color and protects us from UV light damage.

eatrink

- - - - - - - - - - - - - - - - -   the substance our skin produces to make it nearly waterproof and protects us against invading organisms.

ocirenpa

- - - - - - - - - - - - - - - - -   the sweat glands that are located in the groin and armpits and form a thicker form of sweat that produces body odor.

ttarusm

- - - - - - - - - - - - - - - - -   the generic term for the layer of skin in the epidermis.

pillpeaa

- - - - - - - - - - - - - - - - -   "finger-like" structures that connect the dermis to the epidermis of the skin.

CHAPTER 2

Hygiene and Sterilization Techniques

Multiple Choice

Circle the correct answer.

1. Bacteria are
   A. flagellae.
   B. fungi.
   C. viruses.
   D. one-celled microorganisms.

2. Bacteria are classified as
   A. pathogenic and nonpathogenic.
   B. spore and mold.
   C. mycoses and spirilla.
   D. pathogenic and viral.

3. Which one of the two types of bacteria is disease causing?
   A. nonpathogenic
   B. pathogenic
   C. mycoses
   D. viral

4. What are the three types of bacteria?
   A. cocci, flagellae, spirilla
   B. cocci, spirilla, flagellae
   C. bacilli, cocci, spirilla
   D. bacilli, cocci, flagellae

5. The shape of bacilli is
   A. round.
   B. oval.
   C. rodlike.
   D. spiral.

6. The shape of cocci is
   A. round.
   B. rectangular.
   C. rodlike.
   D. spiral.

7. Bacilli can cause
   A. pneumonia.
   B. tetanus.
   C. pustules.
   D. STDs.

8. Spirilla can cause
   A. syphilis.
   B. tuberculosis.
   C. pneumonia.
   D. "strep" throat.

9. Cocci can cause
   A. pustules.
   B. tetanus.
   C. yeast infections.
   D. pneumonia.

10. What happens when bacteria are inactive?
    A. They form cocoon-like shells called spores.
    B. They are easier to kill than when active.
    C. They are likely to morph and change into another type of bacteria.
    D. They form cocoon-like shells called spirillae.

11. Why is the inactive stage especially important?
    A. They are easier to destroy.
    B. Because once they form their shell, called the spore, they are more difficult to kill.
    C. They are more likely to duplicate.
    D. They are more likely to create viral infections.

12. What are two types of fungi?
   A. mold and cocci   B. mildew and bacilli   C. mold and mildew   D. spirillae and mildew

13. What type of fungal infection do we see in humans?
   A. staph   B. strep   C. mycoses   D. TB (tuberculosis)

True/False

Write T for true and F for false in the space provided.

1. ____ Sterilization is the process of killing all microorganisms.

2. ____ An aseptic procedure is the proper handling technique for sterilized equipment.

3. ____ An autoclave is a plastic box with a hole in the top in which you place used lancets and needles.

4. ____ Lancets can be recycled and reused.

5. ____ Disinfectants are chemicals that kill pathogenic microorganisms.

6. ____ Seventy percent isopropyl is not strong enough to kill surface bacteria.

7. ____ Sodium hypochlorite can be used in a 1:10 ratio with water and is a good disinfectant.

8. ____ Performing extractions does not pose any type of cross-contamination issues.

9. ____ Cleaning implements with hot soapy water is adequate for sterilization.

10. ____ A sharps box is a container used for disposing of all used cotton swabs, cleansing pads, and disposable mascara wands.

Fill in the Blank

Using the word bank below, fill in the blank to complete the sentence. The same word may be used more than once.

Word Bank

alcohol	UV sanitizer	autoclave	pumps or flip tops	chlorine bleach
implements	1/2	sodium	gloves	disposable
quaternary ammonium	machine brushes	hypochlorite	OSHA	pumps and tubes
compound	disposable	20 minutes	MSDS	disinfectant

1. Formalin in a 25 percent solution requires that _____ be immersed in solution for at least 10 _____.

2. Mask brushes should be soaked in glutaraldehyde for __ _____.

3. A ___ _____ is a good place for storing disinfected items.

4. _____ _____ should be washed well, then soaked in a disinfectant.

5. High-frequency electrodes should be cleansed and placed in a _____ solution for 20 minutes.

6. _____ in a 70 percent solution requires that implements be immersed for 10 minutes or more for disinfecting.

7. Comedone extractors should be cleansed with 70 percent alcohol, then put in the _____.

8. In a 1:1000 solution, immerse implements for 20 minutes or more using _____ _____ _____.

9. Rinse hands in a ___ percent solution with _____ _____.

10. All cleansing sponges should be _____.

11. When handling soiled laundry or cleaning in general, one should always wear _____.

12. Sheets and towels should be washed with _____ _____.

13. To avoid cross-contamination, the esthetician should always use _____ items for removing creams from jars.

14. _____ __ __ ___ prevent contamination.

15. _____ ___ ____ are best for retail use.

16. _____ is a branch of the federal government that was formed to ensure workplaces provide a safe environment for employees.

17. Special instruction sheets that describe safety concerns of products used in skin-care practices are called _____.

True/False

Write T for true and F for false in the space provided.

1. ____ Bar soap can be used to sanitize hands between client visits.

2. ____ You do not need to wear gloves during procedures.

3. ____ Gloves need to be sterile.

4. ____ You should always start extractions at the chin.

5. ____ Goggles should be worn when performing extractions.

6. ____ Latex gloves are hypoallergenic.

7. ____ You may proceed with a facial on a client with a herpetic breakout as long as you are wearing gloves.

8. ____ You may work on a client if you have an infectious disease as long as you have a mask on.

Define

Use the space provided to define these terms.

1. What are bacteria?

2. Define the term virus.

3. Define sterilization.

4. Define disinfection.

5. What is OSHA?

Word Scramble

Unscramble the key terms below and write the term inside the cells, by using the definitions shown.

neicgoahtp

-------------------   a category of an organism that causes illness and disease.

irailpls

-------------------   a type of bacteria that is spiral in shape—syphilis is the most common disease this form of bacteria causes.

ocicicldpi

-------------------   the smallest type of bacteria that can cause pneumonia or gonorrhea.

osseycm

-------------------   the plural reference to fungus that can cause fungal infections such as Athlete's Foot.

zitanoiilsrte

-------------------   the process of killing all organisms (including inactive bacteria-spores).

Word Puzzle

Just like finding hidden places for organisms to dwell, find the different organisms hidden in this word find. There are ten words. Have fun and happy cleaning!

```
A  G  E  R  M  S  T  Y  M  B  M  T  R  K
D  G  K  U  X  P  P  X  R  X  X  M  N  R
H  E  P  A  T  I  T  I  S  X  E  K  M  X
S  F  E  R  S  R  R  U  A  B  V  Z  X  B
W  X  Y  F  X  I  Q  R  U  T  X  E  K  A
X  X  X  U  X  L  X  X  X  X  P  J  K  C
W  R  I  N  F  L  U  E  N  Z  A  H  E  C
T  E  X  G  X  A  X  T  X  H  T  F  R  I
W  R  X  U  X  X  X  F  Y  X  H  D  X  L
W  E  X  S  T  A  P  H  Y  L  O  C  C  I
Q  P  E  X  Y  X  W  E  R  T  G  U  T  O
X  Y  X  T  X  M  Y  C  O  S  E  S  R  R
Y  T  T  K  R  B  A  X  E  Y  N  Q  D  U
```

CHAPTER 3

The Immune System

Multiple Choice

Circle the correct answer.

1. The body's best mechanism for fighting disease is
   A. the immune system. B. a pathogenic organism. C. the spleen. D. an antibody.

2. A type of bacteria, virus, or other one-celled organism that causes disease is a
   A. nonpathogenic organism. B. antigen. C. pathogenic organism. D. fungus.

3. When you are sick, the process whereby your body builds antibodies to fight disease is called
   A. acquired immunity. B. natural immunity. C. phagocytosis. D. mutation.

4. Polymorphonuclear leukocytes are referred to as
   A. macrophage. B. polymorphs. C. phagocytosis. D. lymphocytes.

5. The process in which polymorphs attack bacteria and other pathogenic organisms is called
   A. macrophage. B. lymphocytes synthesis. C. phagocytosis. D. acquired immunity.

6. The process of white blood cells acting as guards patrolling the body looking for invaders is called
   A. Antigen B. phagocytosis. C. natural immunity. D. lymphocytes.

7. Where is the thymus gland located?
   A. in the thyroid. B. under the arm. C. in the lymph glands. D. under the breastbone in the chest.

8. The function of the thymus gland is to
   A. secrete hormones and trigger synthesis of lymph tissue.　　B. secrete blood cells.

   C. destroy bacteria.　　D. create hormones and destroy bacteria.

9. Two types of lymphocytes are
   A. receptors and T cells. B. receptors and B cells. C. B lymphocytes and T lymphocytes. D. B-killer cells and T-killer cells.

10. B cells make antibodies to prevent further infection or recurrence of disease. They consist of
    A. proteins. B. white blood cells. C. red blood cells. D. lymph tissue.

11. Cell membranes have special communication systems on their surfaces that are called
    A. T-helper cells. B. B lymphocytes. C. receptors. D. T-cell messengers.

12. A hormone type of substance is released by T cells to communicate with one another. It is called
    A. cytoplasm. B. T cell helpers. C. immune system cell. D. interleukin.

13. T cells live approximately
    A. 60 years. B. 25 years. C. 10 years. D. 12 months.

14. Mutation of the cells is created by
    A. one cell duplicating through mitosis. B. several cells changing.
    C. thousands of cells duplicating in the body. D. the immune system killing cells.

15. The term for cancer causing is
    A. mutation. B. carcinogenic. C. oncogenes. D. metastasis.

True/False

Mark T for true and F for false in the space provided.

1. ____ Vaccines are artificial ways of making the immune system produce antibodies.
2. ____ Antibiotics are drugs made from synthetic sources.
3. ____ When cancerous cells divide too fast to be killed by the immune system, cancer develops.
4. ____ Physicians who specialize in the treatment of cancer are called endocrinologists.
5. ____ Because the body is stressed by the repair process while fighting cancerous cells, the immune system is overworked during the rebuilding process.
6. ____ In cancerous cells, the cell membrane is actually the same as the membrane of a normal body cell.
7. ____ Abnormal cell growth can be created by smoking and drinking alcohol.
8. ____ Repeated sun exposure can knock Langerhans cells out of commission long enough to create skin cancer cells.
9. ____ A lack of exercise, overeating, and worry can slow the immune system down, which is called immunosuppression.
10. ____ Too much fat in the diet can create plaque in the blood and obstructs blood flow.

Fill in the Blank

Using the word bank below, fill in the blank to complete the sentence. The same word may be used more than once.

Word Bank

T cells	immune	lymphocytes	metastasis	free radicals
autoimmunity	vaccines	interleukin	natural immunity	subclinical
antibody	antibiotics	carcinogenic	immunosuppression	inflammation
flora	B cells	receptors	plaque	

1. _____ refers to the slowing of the immune system.
2. A buildup of cholesterol and triglycerides in the blood vessels is called _____.
3. Oxygen atoms that are unstable because they have lost an electron in their outer orbit are called ___ _____.
4. _____ _____ is an irritation with no obvious physical symptoms.
5. The "good-guy" type of bacteria is called ____.
6. _____ are located on the surface of the cell membrane to act as a special communication system.
7. When a person possesses the necessary substances and characteristics to avoid contracting a disease he or she is _____.
8. _____ are produced by the lymph nodes, the spleen, and the thymus gland.

9. Drugs made from living organisms are called _____.

10. Substances that cause cancer are _____.

11. _____ is present in the cytoplasm of T cells and released as an alarm system when the T cell is alerted to invasion by a foreign body.

12. A protein produced by the body to help neutralize foreign organisms is called an _____.

13. _ ____ are antibodies made up of proteins that help prevent further infection or recurrence of the disease.

14. _ ____ help alert the immune system to invasion by foreign substances.

15. Immunity to certain diseases present from birth is called a _____ _____.

16. A condition in which the immune system cannot distinguish the difference between antigens and its own cells is called _____.

17. The spreading of cancer is called _____.

18. _____ are artificial ways of making the immune system produce antibodies.

Define, Name, or Detail the Following

1. Name three types of T cells and explain the purpose of each.

   A._____

   B. _____

   C._____

2. Explain what information is located in the DNA of each cell.

   _____

   _____

3. Name three autoimmune diseases.

   A._____

   B. _____

   C._____

4. Name the two forms of lupus and what they each affect.

   A._____

   B. _____

   _____

5. How can we as estheticians help someone with lupus?

   _____

   _____

   _____

   _____

   _____

Word Scramble

Unscramble the key terms below and write the term inside the cells, by using the definitions shown.

myhopcytel

- - - - - - - - - - - - - - - - - is produced in the lymph nodes, the spleen, and the thymus gland.

mnumiloogulnisb

- - - - - - - - - - - - - - - - - or Igs, are antibodies that protect against specific invaders.

intnega

- - - - - - - - - - - - - - - - - refers to a foreign substance recognized by the immune system as an invader.

dyoibtna

- - - - - - - - - - - - - - - - - is a protein that helps neutralize foreign organisms entering the body.

uriedqca ummnityi

- - - - - - - - - - - - - - - - - - is the process of building antibodies to disease when you are sick.

haogycosistp

- - - - - - - - - - - - - - - - - is the process in which polymorphs attack bacteria and other pathogenic organisms.

creoctin

- - - - - - - - - - - - - - - - - tissue is dead tissue.

eghaoprcma

- - - - - - - - - - - - - - - - - is a large type of white blood cell that acts as a guard, constantly patrolling the body looking for foreign invaders.

inescacv

- - - - - - - - - - - - - - - - - are an artificial way of tricking the immune system into making antibodies, or Igs.

urtalan mumiynit

- - - - - - - - - - - - - - - - - is immunity to certain diseases that you have had since you were born.

ticosibitna

- - - - - - - - - - - - - - - - - are drugs made from extracts obtained from living organisms and used to fight bacterial infections.

cida natlem

- - - - - - - - - - - - - - - - - is the layer of lipids and sweat secretions on top of the skin that help kill bacteria.

geranshnal sellc

- - - - - - - - - - - - - - - - - are "guard" cells that constantly patrol the epidermis.

ndrtiesed

- - - - - - - - - - - - - - - - - are tentacle-like structures on the end of some cells including nerves, melanocytes, and Langerhans cells.

sedodopup

- - - - - - - - - - - - - - - - - means "false foot."

ceepotrrs

- - - - - - - - - - - - - - - - - from a specific cell inform T cells of what type of cell the receptor belongs to and that it is an "official" cell of the body and not an antigen.

leuinkerint

- - - - - - - - - - - - - - - - - is present in the cytoplasm of T cells and is released as an alarm system when the T cell is alerted to a foreign body.

atedutm

- - - - - - - - - - - - - - - - - means "changed."

taetsmaiss

- - - - - - - - - - - - - - - - - is the spreading of cancer.

cogolyon

- - - - - - - - - - - - - - - - - is the study of cancer.

Word Puzzle

Just like a microscope can be used to identify different organisms and parts of the immune system that are often too small to be seen with the naked eye, close examination can also show different illnesses that affect the skin. Using your powers of observation, see if you can find terms related to the immune system in the following word search. (*Hint:* the terms are also used in the word scramble above.)

```
N A T U Y A L Y M P H O C Y T E R E N E P L O
I A N U E A L W M P H W C Y T E R E C O P Y B
N L A U M A T I R M U N Y T I R E R P E O M P
T A V I Y X A Y M P H O C Y T E R E O P D P O
E E B U M A L B A U L M R M L Y E T A A O H R
R A O D Y A L B C Y T E V A C C I N E S R O O
A N T I B O D Y U P M V C Y T E M I E P I C E
R T Y L R O D N A T U R A L I M M U N I T Y F
O I Y R A L A U P B V C M E T Y U E E P E T I
R B L O C D I N T E R L E U K I N F C D F E O
K I K R Q Q C Y M N Q O C Y T I O C R P T O R
H O T K U Q L Y U P W O W M U A G C O R O G T
N T J U I A F M A N T I G E N T L T T T P R O
F I T N R Q L Y C P H Q C Y T S O E I O R T P
N C T R E A L Y I Y C P H C O E B Y C D P E M
P S E U D O P O D P H M C Y N S U D O P O D E
G N L U I E Y L M G E A W Y C A L C E D T O T
U E R O M I P H A G O C Y T O S I S C E O I A
D A E M M A L B N P H R C A L T N I O N I C S
G A C M U S A L T V P O N C O I S B O D I C T
B A E U N A W B L P W P C N G L G Y E R T O A
A D P A I D L W E A B H U G Y E O L G I I T S
M U T A T E D B S P H A C B A C I C O T I C I
P A O M Y L B P L A N G E R H A N S C E L L S
S D R P B A M A W P B E U N A L T B E S T O P
E E S U M A L B A U L M R M L Y E T A A O H R
```

CHAPTER 4

Communicable Diseases

Multiple Choice

Circle the correct answer.

1. Communicable diseases
   A. are rarely curable.

   C. are not preventable.

   B. are not devastating for the most part and are easily curable.

   D. do not spread that easily.

2. Estheticians should be able to recognize diseases so that
   A. they may refer the client to a doctor for treatment.

   C. they can protect themselves from contracting the disease.

   B. they may be better able to treat the client.

   D. they may be able to give better advice to the client about how to treat the disease.

3. Infectious diseases
   A. are highly contagious diseases and can be easily transferred by contaminated hands or skin-care implements.

   C. are usually obvious.

   B. are always dangerous and can be debilitating.

   D. have a long recovery period.

4. Conjunctivitis is a bacterial disease of the
   A. skin.   B. eye.   C. finger.   D. foot.

5. The esthetician should work on a client with conjunctivitis
   A. with personal protective devices.

   C. never.

   B. with gloves on.

   D. for treatments only, no makeup.

6. Herpes simplex is a
   A. bacterial infection.   B. fungus.   C. virus.   D. condition that affects the hands.

7. Impetigo is a
   A. disorder that affects primarily adults.

   C. condition that occurs mostly on the feet.

   B. bacterial infection that is most often seen in children but can be spread to adults.

   D. viral infection that is characterized by crusty lesions that ooze or weep.

8. The number one risk for contracting HIV infection is
   A. kissing.

   C. having sexual intercourse.

   B. touching unclean surfaces.

   D. living with someone with HIV.

9. No one actually dies of AIDS; they die of
   A. infections and diseases.   B. HIV.

   C. diseases and contamination.   D. dehydration and fluid in the lungs.

10. To diagnose an HIV infection as AIDS, a person must be
    A. feeling some symptoms.   B. not sexually active for several weeks.

    C. HIV positive.   D. in the window phase.

True/False

Mark T for true and F for false in the space provided.

1. ____ An esthetician can work on a client with conjunctivitis.

2. ____ Methicillin-resistant *Staphylococcus aureus* (MRSA) is a bacterium that easily responds to antibiotics.

3. ____ Impetigo can show up anywhere on the skin.

4. ____ Herpes simplex is managed with antiviral drugs.

5. ____ The hepatitis virus can live quietly in the liver after symptoms have gone away.

6. ____ Hepatitis can live on a surface for up to 1 week.

7. ____ Technically, hepatitis viruses are harder to kill than HIV and are much more numerous in body fluids.

8. ____ There is still no cure for AIDS.

9. ____ Some of the last symptoms of HIV infection or AIDS show up on the skin.

10. ____ The window phase is the period of time between exposure to HIV and the time antibodies are made.

Matching

Match the term with the best description, and write the letter of the term in the space provided.

Description   *Terms*

1. ____ A tumor-like eruption that occurs on the tongue or   A. monogamous
   the insides of the cheeks.

2. ____ A yellowing of the skin and eyes, abdominal pain, fever,   B. hepatitis
   and constant fatigue.

3. ____ Two persons who engage in sex, are faithful to one another,   C. oral thrush
   and never have sex with another person.

4. ____ An injury of a health-care worker by accidentally being stuck   D. abstinent people
   with a used or dirty needle from a patient with HIV.

5. ____ A yeast infection of the mouth.   E. herpes

6. ____ A virus that comes in many forms.   F. hairy leukoplakia

7. ____ Persons who do not engage in sexual intercourse at all.   G. jaundice

8. ____ An inflammation of the liver caused by a viral infection.   H. needle-stick injury

Short Answer

1. The esthetician should not attempt to _____ ____, or give advice to clients about diseases.

2. _____ _____ are highly contagious diseases that can easily be transferred by contaminated hands or skin-care implements.

3. Viruses work by _____ themselves into healthy cells.

4. _____ _____ _____ _____ is a syndrome caused by a virus known as _____ _____ ____.

5. Two types of blood tests are able to isolate the HIV antibody. The first is called the _____ test. Confirmation is accomplished with a second test called the _____ ___ test.

6. _____ _____ help restore (or partially restore) the immune system.

7. _____ helps prevent people from getting a disease.

8. Name the five different types of hepatitis, and give a brief description of each.

    A._____

    _____

    B._____

    _____

    C._____

    _____

    D._____

    _____

    E._____

    _____

9. List seven myths about AIDS.

    A._____

    _____

    B._____

    _____

    C._____

    _____

    D._____

    _____

    E._____

    _____

    F._____

    _____

    G._____

    _____

Define

Use the space provided to define these terms.

1. HIV:

_____

_____

_____

_____

_____

2. Window phase:

_____

_____

_____

_____

3. Opportunistic infections:

_____

_____

_____

_____

_____

4. Dementia:

_____

_____

_____

_____

5. Enzyme inhibitors:

_____

_____

_____

_____

_____

Word Scramble

Unscramble the key terms below and write the term inside the cells, by using the definitions shown.

encenistba

- - - - - - - - - - - - - - - - -   means that the persons do not engage in sexual intercourse at all.

rpeseh

- - - - - - - - - - - - - - - - -   refers to a group of viruses.

erseph soretz

- - - - - - - - - - - - - - - - -   is the virus that causes both shingles and chickenpox.

lesinghs

- - - - - - - - - - - - - - - - -   known also as herpes zoster, is caused by the same virus, varicella zoster that causes chickenpox.
The lesions of herpes zoster look like multiple red blisters.

arstw

- - - - - - - - - - - - - - - - -   are caused by a variety of viruses known as papovavirus or verruca.

mucslluom tanocgisomu

- - - - - - - - - - - - - - - - -   is a viral infection frequently seen on the faces of children; it appears as groups of small, flesh-colored
papules.

eptiogmi

- - - - - - - - - - - - - - - - -   is a skin infection characterized by large, open, weeping lesions.

soseymc

- - - - - - - - - - - - - - - - -   are fungal infections.

culiitsillof

- - - - - - - - - - - - - - - - -   is a bacterial infection of the hair follicle.

orhricebes matitisred

- - - - - - - - - - - - - - - - -   or seborrhea, is an inflammation of the sebaceous glands and follicles resulting in redness, flaking,
and itching in oily areas of the face.

arol rushth

- - - - - - - - - - - - - - - - -   is an infection of the mouth and throat caused by the yeast known as *Candida albicans.*

yirha oplkaiaukel

- - - - - - - - - - - - - - - - -   is a tumor-like eruption that can occur on the tongue or the insides of the cheeks.

opsiak's comarsa

- - - - - - - - - - - - - - - - -   is a rare form of skin cancer characterized by purple-brown lesions.

titsiaphe

- - - - - - - - - - - - - - - - -   is an inflammation of the liver.

sishorirc

- - - - - - - - - - - - - - - - -   is scarring within the liver caused by chronic inflammation; it can be caused by chronic viral infection
and is often caused by alcoholism. This can lead to liver failure, liver cancer, and death.

unicdeja

- - - - - - - - - - - - - - - - -   is a yellowing of the skin and eyes.

Word Puzzle

Just like a microscope can be used to identify different organisms that cause communicable disease, such as HIV, or different hepatitis viruses that are often too small to be seen with the naked eye, close examination can also often show illnesses that affect the skin. Using your powers of observation, see if you can find terms related to communicable disease in the following word search. (*Hint:* the terms are also used in the word scramble above.)

```
S E B O O R R H E I C O D E R M S A K I T R S S H M
P R E R K O H F I A S H I N G L E S A K L R T I Z R
S A H A R R K M P X C Q U M M M B J P K M X X D G M
M O L L U S C U M C O N T A G I O S U M D L T Z D R
D K F T E M K R P Q C M Y C C O R E S N L N I O K R
A F L H O P L O F D Q E G N H Q R J I L I M Y P A A
S A H R R R K M P X C Q M U E M H J X D K M X D P M
P F K U P O L N F W Q W H E R P E S K S L L H T O Z
D C I S R H O S I S Q U M J P A I M L N E O R T S R
A F L H P O L O H F E Q G Q E B C J S L M R P A I A
E E R O O K H N I O A D Y U S O D A M Y C O S E S Z
R A H R R K M G X L C Q U N Z M E J C K M S D T S M
P F K P O L N L W L Q W E D O N R K O L H L Z T A Z
E E B O R R H E I I C I D I S R M A M I A T Z S R M
S E M O L L U C S C U M C N T O A B S T I N E N C E
E S N L N I O J A U N D I C E R T E E R R O Z K O N
L M R P A R A M P L Q A U P R N I P F K Y Z O P M K
M L N E O R T E R I U W M R N T T U M C L E E R A T
J C K M S D T M S T M A L E O C I T L P E O R T E P
A F L P O L O F C I R R H O S I S J T L U M R P A A
D F O L L C I C U S I T T I S M M J N T K N E O Q R
S A H R K R P M P X C S P I M P E T I G O M S D S M
H E P A T T I S I S C O D A R S A I A S P T P S L M
T P S L M H E P A T I S I S C O D S A R L A F L P O
M R P A A E S N L N I O T I S M M J N T A S C O D A
J P K M X X D G M E E R O O K H N I T I K H E P A T
I C O D E R M A K I T R S S H H E P A T I T I S M R
J S L M R P A P A J P K M X X D G M E E A R T P S L
```

CHAPTER 5

Hormones

Multiple Choice

Circle the correct answer.

1. Hormones are
   A. located primarily in the sebaceous glands and are the cause of acne.
   B. special chemicals that are manufactured or secreted by glands within the body.
   C. glands that create sebaceous and sudoriferous activity.
   D. located on cell membranes that are like "locks" whereby "keys" or specific hormones affect the cell in different ways.

2. Estheticians need to be familiar with hormones because
   A. they will need to advise clients and patients on the type and amount they should be taking.
   B. hormones have definite effects on the skin, and their functioning is directly related to many skin problems.
   C. hormones are easily controlled once you understand their primary function.
   D. hormones are responsible for 90 percent of all skin problems.

3. Exocrine glands
   A. are present in the groin and underarm areas.
   B. secrete hormones.
   C. are glands such as the sebaceous and sudoriferous glands.
   D. are present in the center of the head.

4. Endocrine glands
   A. are located in the center of the brain.
   B. are found in the groin and underarms.
   C. secrete hormones directly into the bloodstream.
   D. work by transmitting chemical messengers to the various body cells.

5. Apocrine glands are present in the
   A. groin and underarm areas.
   B. center of the brain, the pituitary.
   C. sebaceous glands.
   D. sex hormones.

6. There are "keys" that fit "locks," causing the cell membrane to produce enzymes that stimulate other chemical reactions within the cell. Those locks are called
   A. receptors.   B. secretors.   C. transmitters.   D. receivers.

7. How many major endocrine glands are located in the body?
   A. 4   B. 3   C. 2   D. 8

8. The pituitary gland secretes many hormones called
   A. adrenal.   B. estrogen.   C. trophic.   D. testosterone.

9. The "signal" hormones that are responsible for causing glands to make hormones are called
   A. trophic hormones.   B. sex hormones.   C. androgens.   D. FSH.

10. The hypothalamus gland
    A. is directly responsible for creating hormones.
    B. creates chemicals that cause other glands to make hormones.
    C. controls some involuntary muscles, such as the muscles of the intestines that help move material through the gastrointestinal system.
    D. informs T cells of what type it is, and whether it is an "official" cell of the body and not an antigen.

11. A hormone specialist is called
    A. an endocrinologist.   B. an oncologist.   C. a nephrologist.   D. an internist.

True/False

Mark T for true and F for false in the space provided.

1. ____ Sex glands are found in the center of the head, in the pituitary.

2. ____ The hypothalamus, an endocrine gland, is connected to the brain or pituitary gland where it controls some involuntary muscles such as those in the intestine.

3. ____ Trophic hormones are chemicals that cause other glands to make signal hormones.

4. ____ FSH (follicle-stimulating hormone) allows production of sex hormones in the glands present in the organs.

5. ____ The thymus is located in the neck; it regulates both cellular and body metabolism and produces hormones that stimulate growth.

6. ____ Thyroxine is responsible for regulating calcium and phosphates in the bloodstream necessary for proper bone growth.

7. ____ The adrenal glands are located just above the kidneys, and they produce two hormones needed by the nervous system to transport nerve impulses.

8. ____ The pineal gland is located in the brain and is theorized to be related to the sex hormones.

9. ____ The islets of Langerhans are located in the abdomen; they secrete enzymes that are delivered into the intestines and help digest foods.

10. ____ The thymus produces specialized lymphocytes to help the body fight disease.

Matching

Match the term with the best description, and write the letter of the term in the space provided.

Description	Terms
1. The stage of life when physical changes occur in both sexes and when sexual function of the sex glands begins to take place is __.	A. ovaries and testes
2. Usually at about 12 to 14 years of age the hypothalamus begins producing a hormone called __, which in turn stimulates the pituitary gland to produce larger amounts of FSH and LH.	B. androgens
3. FSH and LH cause the __ to secrete hormones, estrogens and androgens.	C. puberty
4. At this time the sebaceous glands produce more __.	D. luteinizing hormone
5. __ are responsible for creating more sebum, which in turn creates a dilation of the follicles.	E. sebum
6. The nose is the first area to develop __.	F. keratosis pilaris
7. __ should be taught to preteens and teenagers.	G. estrogen and progesterone

8. __ is a skin condition often seen at puberty, which presents as small pinpoint bumps that can be accompanied by redness.

9. During the six stages of the menstrual cycle __ are periodically adjusted.

10. Premenstrual syndrome is accompanied by __.

11. __ is often associated with the hormonal activity during PMS (premenstrual syndrome).

12. Some __ may cause acne flares.

13. During pregnancy __, or pregnancy mask, can develop.

14. __, or lightening agents, should never be used on pregnant women (or while lactating/breastfeeding) for hyperpigmentation or melasma.

15. Stretch marks, or __, also occur in pregnant women.

16. __ created during pregnancy are caused by an increase in blood flow and blood pressure. They are characterized by small, red, enlarged capillaries on the face and other parts of the body.

17. __ is the phase that is prior to menopause.

18. The drop in hormone levels in the bloodstream can cause __.

19. __ should not be used by women in whom there is a history of breast cancer in the immediate family.

20. Acne flare-ups can be caused by __ at any age.

H. larger follicle openings/ pores

I. birth control methods

J. home care compliance

K. hot flashes

L. mood swings

M. chin acne

N. striae

O. melasma

P. hydroquinone

Q. telangiectases

R. perimenopause

S. hormone fluctuations

T. hormone replacement therapy

Fill in the Blank

Using the word bank below, fill in the blank to complete the sentence. The same word may be used more than once.

Word Bank

facial swelling	galvanic/high	alpha hydroxy acids	hyperpigmentation	hormone replacement
hot flashes	frequency	(AHAs)	formication	therapy (HRT)
flare-up	massage	improve	hirsutism	perimenopausal
patch test		acne	rapidly growing nails	

1. Among many treatments and products contraindicated for pregnancy, _____ _____ are two that estheticians should never perform on pregnant women without written permission from a physician.

2. A _____ ___ should always be performed on pregnant women prior to fully waxing an area to avoid irritation and unusual reaction to the treatment.

3. For a client struggling with PMS, a _____ could provide the best treatment for calming and soothing.

4. ____ _____ ____ _____ have not been fully studied enough to prove safe for pregnant women.

5. PMS can cause a _____.

6. A type of birth control pill that contains estrogen and progesterone can cause acne-prone skin to _____.

7. A type of birth control pill that contains high levels of progesterone can cause acne-prone skin to _____.

8. Birth control methods can create _____.

9. _____ often is the phase associated with many of the symptoms that have been considered menopausal.

10. A drop in hormone levels can create a variety of symptoms in women such as ___ _____, rapid heart beat, emotional irritability, vaginal dryness, and bloating.

11. The use of _____ _____ _____ _____ is currently being reevaluated for use during menopause, and the decision to use it should be carefully considered based on personal and family history, symptoms and their severity, and a thorough consultation with a qualified physician.

12. _____ is an itching and tingling feeling of the skin experienced by some women during menopause.

13. To avoid ___ _____ or undue distress, it is important to not use too much heat during the treatment of menopausal women.

14. _____ is excessive hair growth.

15. A woman who is obese may experience hormonal fluctuation that may show up on the skin as ____.

16. Hyperthyroidism is a condition in which the thyroid gland produces too much thyroid hormone, and a person with hyperthyroidism may exhibit symptoms such as _____ _____ ____.

17. ____ _____ may be present on a client with hypothyroidism.

Define, Name, or Detail the Following

1. Name eight menopausal symptoms.

   A. _____

   B. _____

   C. _____

   D. _____

   E. _____

   F. _____

   G. _____

   H. _____

2. Define hyperthyroidism.

   _____

   _____

   _____

3. Define hypothyroidism.

   _____

   _____

   _____

4. Name the major endocrine glands.

   _____

   _____

   _____

5. Detail the precautions an esthetician should take when treating pregnant women.

   _____

   _____

   _____

Word Scramble

Unscramble the key terms below and write the term inside the cells, by using the definitions shown.

mosenorh

- - - - - - - - - - - - - - - - -   are special chemicals that are manufactured or secreted by glands within the body.

redetecs

- - - - - - - - - - - - - - - - -   means synthesized or released by various cells or organs.

rineocex andslg

- - - - - - - - - - - - - - - - -   such as the sebaceous glands and the sudoriferous glands have ducts through which chemicals move.

pocinrea landsg

- - - - - - - - - - - - - - - - -   are present in the groin area and armpits. They produce a thicker form of sweat and are responsible for producing the substance that, when in contact with bacteria, produces body odor.

nriencode andlgs

- - - - - - - - - - - - - - - - -   secrete hormones directly into the bloodstream.

ecepotrsr

- - - - - - - - - - - - - - - - -   inform T cells about the type of cell it is and that it is an "official" cell of the body and not an antigen.

ituptiray dnagl

- - - - - - - - - - - - - - - - -   is found in the center of the head. It serves as the "brain" of the endocrine system.

pothyhlaamus ndalg

- - - - - - - - - - - - - - - - -   controls some involuntary muscles, such as the muscles of the intestines that help move food through the gastrointestinal system.

rohroonmseuen

- - - - - - - - - - - - - - - - -   are secreted by the hypothalamus and trigger the pituitary gland to make specific hormones.

pohtalaumsyh

- - - - - - - - - - - - - - - - -   manufactures hormones that stimulate the pituitary gland to make other hormones. It is also able to detect needs of various parts of the body by chemically monitoring the blood.

opichrt ormonesh

- - - - - - - - - - - - - - - - -   are chemicals that cause other glands to make hormones.

yriodth langd

- - - - - - - - - - - - - - - - -   is located in the neck. It regulates both cellular and body metabolism and produces hormones that stimulate growth.

roinxeyth

- - - - - - - - - - - - - - - - -   is one of the two main hormones secreted by the thyroid gland.

oninticcal

- - - - - - - - - - - - - - - - -   is one of the hormones secreted by the thyroid gland.

yoidrhatrap glnda

- - - - - - - - - - - - - - - - -   is responsible for regulating calcium and phosphates in the bloodstream.

ardenla sandgl

- - - - - - - - - - - - - - - - -   are located just above the kidneys and produce hormones needed by the nervous system to transport nerve impulses.

enainelrda

- - - - - - - - - - - - - - - - -   is secreted when the body is under stress.

piealn nadgl

- - - - - - - - - - - - - - - - -   is located in the brain. Its function is not well understood, but it is theorized to be related to the sex hormones.

(continued)

pcarnesa

-----------------   is located in the abdomen. It secretes pancreatic enzymes that are delivered into the intestine.

iabested

-----------------   is a disease that results from the pancreas not secreting enough insulin.

msuyht gldna

-----------------   is located under the breastbone in the chest. It secretes hormones and helps trigger synthesis of more lymph tissue.

oarisev

-----------------   are located just above the uterus and are connected to the uterus by two hollow tubes called fallopian tubes.

estest

-----------------   are present within the scrotum and produce sperm.

osterenotset

-----------------   is the male hormone responsible for development of typical male characteristics.

roegnsdna

-----------------   are male hormones.

Word Puzzle

Just like a microscope can be used to identify different organisms that cause communicable disease, such as HIV, or different hepatitis viruses that are often too small to be seen with the naked eye, close examination can also show different illnesses that affect the skin. See if you can find terms related to communicable disease by examining the words in the following word search. (*Hint:* the terms are also used in the word scramble above.)

```
P C R S O E A S N B O C R P N E D G L A N D S N L M H N E S
P N N C R E A P I W T U I T A R Y G L A N D S N L S Y N E D
E P A P I R E A A N D O C P R N E D G L A N D S P L P M N Q
X B C R D E W A N R Y O C A D N E D G L A N S N I Q O H E C
O V A R I E S A T N D O C N T H Y M U S G P L A N D T R Y W
C I P C A A N I E E W A N C A L C I T O N I N G E A H D Q E
R C O I B B C R S R E A A R N D O C R E I T S G A G A R P Q
I I C E E R E A T P E A M E N A C C H E A U S Z L C L R A N
N E R A T H Y R O I D G L A N D R E A A H I E A G Z A C R R
E A I N E B Q X S E D R C S I E E D G I A T S N L M M M A E
G E N A S A N M T A R B Q X H A R B Q X C A L N A C U N T N
L R E A R B Q X E A A N T R O P H I C H O R M O N E S C H N
A N G M S M N Q R I E E D G R D O C R N E Y D A D A G A Y A
N R L R E H Y P O T H A L A M U S I E E D G G I A D L A R I
D N A L D M N D N P N D I R O D A L N N E L D N L G A D O G
S A N A M M I R E M A D R E N A L I N E S A S N D S N S I S
E A D R E A E T A R B Q X A E A H Z C U A N I A A I D A D Z
M N S P A N Q H Q T E S T E S D N O V R A D L N N E M M G E
L S M N Q T G Y L A N E D D G L A L N O D N L G D D D G L N
P A A I R H E M A A N C D O C R N E D H E D G I R L P M A E
A R B Q X Y A U E D R R I E E D G I A O S N D S O S N D N M
G R N E D R L S N D S E L D M N Q A D R E N A L G L A N D S
L A C C M O A G T A D T C R D N O V A M I E S N E N G G E A
D A N C R X W L A S T E D R E C E P T O R S A N N S N E M M
I A A C R I A A N D I D R G T E D G E N N B S T S L P M M E
A N S N D N F N F E M S M A N S N D N E P D N W R A N S N D
P A A W R E N D O C R I N E G L A N D S A N S N D S M M F E
```

CHAPTER 6

Skin Analysis

Multiple Choice

Circle the correct answer.

1. From the esthetician's perspective a skin analysis is
   A. the process of determining the client's skin type and conditions that require esthetic care.
   B. the process of specific problems with the skin.
   C. the process of determining the client's Fitzpatrick skin type.
   D. the process of looking at specific treatments for the client.

2. Dr. Thomas Fitzpatrick created the Fitzpatrick Skin Typing system to determine
   A. the type of skin a client has.
   B. the amount of sun damage a client has and what it needs to improve.
   C. the tolerance of different skin types to the sun's burning rays.
   D. the color of the skin when it tans.

3. The Fitzpatrick Skin Typing system is helpful to estheticians because
   A. it makes the skin analysis process easier.
   B. it provides the esthetician with a guide to determine potential reaction and tolerance for facial treatments, products, and ingredients that may be selected for the client.
   C. it provides a guide to determine whether a person should use antioxidants.
   D. it provides a tool to determine whether a client should use a sunscreen.

4. When looking at the Fitzpatrick scale, a Type 1 is
   A. fair skinned with light-brown hair and green eyes and prone to burning.
   B. fair skinned with blond or red hair, prone to burning, then tans.
   C. fair skinned with blond or red hair, prone to burning, and never tans.
   D. fair skinned with blond or red hair and tans easily.

5. A Type IV on the Fitzpatrick scale is
   A. medium-brown skin, brown eyes, tans and gets darker easily.
   B. darker skin with black-brown eyes, burns slightly, and then gets tan.
   C. medium-brown skin, light hair and eyes, gets dark tan.
   D. medium-brown skin, lighter eyes, tans minimally.

6. It is important for the esthetician to take a full health history on a client because
   A. the esthetician needs to know if the client has been ill recently.
   B. it will give the esthetician information about what the client is currently using.
   C. it will give the esthetician information about what they are interested in pursuing.
   D. it will give the esthetician information about the client, his or her habits, medical conditions, and information that can affect your treatment of the client's skin.

7. Contraindications are
    A. treatments that you can use under very extreme conditions.

    B. treatment techniques, procedures, products, or ingredients that must be avoided as a result of individual client conditions that may cause side effects or somehow endanger client's health.

    C. pregnancy, pacemakers, epilepsy, high blood pressure, and any other health problems that you may be concerned about while treating a client.

    D. treatment techniques that are indicated for use but only if following MSDS standards.

8. Which of the following is the general rule for working with a client who has a medical condition?
    A. If you have treated a client with the same type of condition before and you have experience with the condition, you may provide treatment.

    B. If you have experience treating clients with various conditions, you will be able to recognize problems as they arise.

    C. If you have any doubt about treating a client with medical conditions, check with the client's physician prior to treating the client.

    D. If you have any doubt about treating a client with problems, refer to the most current reference material on the topic and contact your supervisor.

9. Skin conditions are
    A. often treatable disorders of the skin and can be improved with esthetic treatment.

    B. rarely treatable and need medical care.

    C. usually the result of neglect.

    D. often caused by overexfoliating.

10. Vehicles are
    A. usually used to hydrate the skin.

    B. used to provide the carrying base and spreading agent of a product.

    C. used in a product to transport ingredients to correct unwanted conditions.

    D. used to provide exfoliation to skin that is struggling with acne.

True/False

Mark T for true and F for false in the space provided.

1. ____ If a client has a medical condition, the esthetician may treat the client if the appropriate steps have been taken to assure the client's health and safety.

2. ____ Skin types are related to the amount of sebum being produced by the sebaceous glands.

3. ____ Skin conditions are rarely treatable through esthetic treatment and skin-care products.

4. ____ The analysis procedure always begins with cleansing the skin.

5. ____ After establishing the skin type during the analysis procedure, you may observe medical conditions that should always be referred to a physician.

6. ____ A normal skin type will have clean pores, but they will be of varied sizes.

7. ____ Oily skin will always exhibit breakouts and may have some small pores on the chin.

8. ____ Dry skin will exhibit very small pores (nearly invisible) and may be dehydrated.

9. ____ Closed comedones present as small, white bumps just under the skin surface.

10. ____ Sebaceous hyperplasias look like a daisy or donut, are caused by an overgrowth of sebaceous glands, and are often indicative of oily and sun-damaged areas.

11. ____ Milia are characterized by "open pores" or ice pick scars; these are small scarred follicles that always appear enlarged.

12. ____ Rhytides are smoother areas on the skin that require hydration.

Short Answer

1. _____ is a lack of firmness and elasticity.

2. A rough texture to the touch is considered _____ _____.

3. A European esthetic term referring to enlarged pore structure in older sun-damaged skin is _____.

4. _____ is characterized by sun-related freckles, splotches, or hyperpigmentation.

5. Skin that is red with oily skin symptoms is often classified as _____.

6. Dilated red capillaries are _____.

7. _____ is the medical term for redness.

8. A medical condition characterized by redness in the nasal region, cheeks, and sometimes forehead and chin is called _____.

9. _____ is overproduction of melanin resulting in dark splotches.

10. A lack of melanin in an area is called _____.

11. Freckles caused by sun exposure are called _____.

12. Pigmentation problems can affect any _____.

13. _____ is a medical condition resulting in absence of pigment in areas.

14. "Pregnancy mask" is known as _____.

15. _____ _____ _____ is characterized by dark-pigmented areas related to some type of trauma, such as pigmentation left from acne blemishes, chronic picking at acne lesions, or overtreating skin with a high melanin content.

Define

Use the space provided to define these terms.

1. Normal skin

_____

_____

_____

2. Oily skin

_____

_____

_____

3. Dry/alipidic skin

_____

_____

_____

4. Combination skin/oily

_____

_____

_____

5. Combination skin/dry

_____

_____

_____

6. Birthmarks

_____

_____

_____

7. Port-wine stains

_____

_____

_____

8. Charting

_____

_____

_____

9. Client confidentiality

_____

_____

_____

_____

Word Scramble

Unscramble the key terms below and write the term inside the cells, by using the definitions shown.

ctaoinscotnarnidi

------------------ are treatment techniques, products, or ingredients that must be avoided because of individual client conditions that may cause side effects or possibly endanger the client's health.

evihlecs

------------------ are the spreading agents in skin-care or cosmetic products.

rope

------------------ is the lay term for *follicle*, it is most often used in referring to the top view of the follicle.

etermprei

------------------ is the outside edge of the face, bordered by the ears, lower chin and neck, and top of the forehead.

rnigtahc

------------------ is the process of creating a written record of clinical observations and treatments in a client's or patient's chart.

pertyhrohicp

------------------ describes a raised scar above the skin's surface.

trohicpophy

------------------ describes a depressed scar.

arkmkpco

------------------ is a hypotrophic scar often caused by chicken pox or acne.

schmorisayd

------------------ are conditions that cause changes in the normal colors of the skin.

tniirnics ingga

------------------ sometimes referred to as natural aging, is aging of the skin due to genetics, gravity, and other factors that people have no control over.

osistsale

------------------ is lack of skin firmness and lack of elasticity.

draionthyed

------------------ is a condition in which the skin lacks moisture in the surface cells.

tisedyrh

------------------ are wrinkles.

Word Puzzle

Just like examining skin for type and condition, looking for things and textures can be valuable—even if it is a silly word game. See if you can find terms related to skin condition and type in the following word search. (*Hint:* the terms are also used in the word scramble above.)

```
T N S G N T D R A V R N V I A A T U O N S N V I
H Y R H N P Y E I R I M T E T E R E M T O R H D
T F T H T K S K R A A R N H R H H A T O A O G Y
H H T Y P O C P R O P T H I C O X A T W P O W S
T N T T H H H I R A I C N C W H D E O Q E D H C
H T Y I O G R O R A L T N L N Q F J E N R O W H
H N D N N T O P O H Y P E R T R O P H I C E F R
Y Y E O J T M R O Y H I N S I K H O Y N L K G O
P N C S J H I P R P F N D I J P D W W T A W P M
D E H Y D R A T I O N H H T Y P O H N R T N S G
P N A S J H S P R T C F N D I J V E H I C L E S
E T R S M N Q R K R F N D F K W R X Y N T S Q I
R N T S O H T R P O R E N D E L W A F S T W A F
S O I Y Y E O J T P H N D N I R H Y T I D E S T
F N N O R A L T N H Y Y E P T N T T H C H L S G
H H G T N T T H H I H T Y E H H T Y P A W A T N
S I K H O Y K P O C K M A R K T N T T G T S W H
T N L N Q F J E N R O W H I I J P D W I W T P N
T E R E M T O R H D S I K M H T W A F N H O W A
C W H D E O Q E D H C T E E Y Y E O J G T S O J
W C O N T R A I N D I C A T I O N S E O J I T N
H I C O X A T W P O W S H E T N L N Q F N S F N
R N V I A A T U O N S N V R H H T Y P O H N T Y
```

CHAPTER 7

Recognize and Refer Medical Conditions

Multiple Choice

Circle the correct answer.

1. The esthetician should be trained to
   A. diagnose common skin diseases and disorders.

   C. treat most common skin ailments and refer to a dermatologist only as a last resort.

   B. recognize common medical conditions and diseases and refer them to the proper medical authority, in most cases a dermatologist.

   D. calm the client if something suspicious is suspected.

2. A lesion is
   A. any mark on the skin that is not a normal part of the skin.

   C. an open wound.

   B. an area of red splotches.

   D. a hyperpigmented area.

3. Primary lesions
   A. are the smallest.

   C. need to be removed.

   B. are uniform in nature.

   D. are lesions that are in the earliest stages of development.

4. Macules are
   A. flat (nonelevated) marks on the skin in which there is only a change in the normal color of the skin.

   C. lesions that are considered tumors.

   B. papules that are raised areas on the skin that are generally smaller than 1 centimeter.

   D. large vesicles.

5. A wheal is a
   A. blister.   B. hive.   C. scale.   D. scab.

6. Erosion refers to
   A. any area of redness that appears to be scaling.

   C. a shallow depression in the skin.

   B. purpura.

   D. a raised area in the skin.

7. Atrophy means
   A. hypertrophy.

   C. building up of tissue.

   B. wasting away, a loss of tissue.

   D. a linear lesion.

8. Keratosis is
   A. a thinning of the epidermis

   C. a scaly, patchy area.

   B. any area with less pigment.

   D. a thickening of the stratum corneum.

9. A serpiginous lesion is a
   A. mole.   B. nonpigmented lesion.   C. ring-shaped lesion.   D. lesion with a snake-like pattern.

10. Eczematization refers to
   A. a combination of symptoms, including erythema, weeping, vesicles, and crusting.
   B. a combination of symptoms, such as hyperpigmentation, erythema, keratosis, and purpura.
   C. a shallow depression in the skin that presents in a round pattern.
   D. lentigines that are multiple sizes and colors.

True/False

Mark T for true and F for false in the space provided.

1. ____ Impetigo is a bacterial skin infection that is commonly seen on the face but can appear anywhere, and which is characterized by large, open, weeping lesions.

2. ____ Folliculitis is a viral infection.

3. ____ Cellulitis is a deep infection of the dermis caused by streptococcus.

4. ____ Erysipelas is a severe form of bacterial cellulitis.

5. ____ Tinea versicolor is sometimes called "sun fungus."

6. ____ Tinea corporis is commonly known as "athlete's foot."

7. ____ Fungal infections are called mycoses.

8. ____ Herpes refers to a group of viruses.

9. ____ Chemical peels may help a client with an active herpetic breakout.

10. ____ Molluscum contagiosum is a viral infection that appears as groups of small, flesh-colored papules.

Fill in the Blank

Using the word bank below, fill in the blank to complete the sentence. The same word may be used more than once.

Word Bank

dermatitis	herpes zoster	psoriasis	milia	skin tags
contact dermatitis	atopic	urticaria	couperose	xanthomas
warts	dermatitis/eczema	keratosis pilaris		

1. _____ ____ is known as shingles and is caused by the same virus that causes chicken pox.

2. An irritation caused by an allergic reaction or irritation to something or some substance touching the skin or coming in contact with the skin's surface is _____ _____.

3. ____ are caused by a variety of viruses known as papovaviruses or verrucae.

4. Inflammation of the skin is known as _____.

5. A chronic inflammatory condition of the skin that is hereditary and may be related to respiratory allergies or asthma is called ____ _____.

6. ____ ___ are very small, thread-like growths that present commonly on the eyelids, neck, and décolleté.

7. Fatty pockets located on the eyelids are called _____.

8. Hives or an outbreak of _____ is the result of allergies.

9. An inflammatory disorder of the skin caused by the skin and epidermis "turning over" faster than it does under normal conditions is called _____.

10. A condition in which the skin is exhibiting redness and irritation patches, accompanied by a rough texture and small pinpoint white papules that look like small milia is known as _____ ____.

11. Small white deposits of sebum between the follicle and the corneum are called _____.

12. "Broken capillaries" have been called _____ by estheticians; they are considered vascular lesions or telangiectases.

Short Answer

1. Renova®, Retin-A®, Avita®, Differin®, and Tazorac® are all examples of _____ ____.

2. These drugs cause ____ _____ of the skin, which can cause _____, _____, redness, and _____.

3. _____ is an oral drug used for the treatment of ____. There are many side effects associated with its use, and the client/patient must be followed closely by his or her physician.

4. Female patients undergoing treatment for acne with _____ are required to use ____ _____.

5. Two other drugs that are used to treat acne, rosacea, sun damage, and hyperpigmentation are _____ and _____.

6. A drug that is used to treat melasma and hyperpigmentation is called _____. It is a combination of _____, _____, and _____ _____ _____.

7. _____ is a prescription-strength skin lightener (usually at 4 percent concentration) used to treat hyperpigmentation.

8. Drugs for the treatment of rosacea are:

   A. _____

   B. _____

   C. _____

   D. _____

9. _____ is a hormone (steroid) that helps relieve inflammation, redness, and other skin irritations.

10. Chronic use of _____ may cause _____ of the skin.

Define

Use the space provided to define these terms.

1. Abscess

   _____

   _____

2. Vesicle

   _____

   _____

3. Lentigines

   _____

   _____

4. Erythema

   _____

   _____

5. Hypopigmentation

   _____

   _____

Word Scramble

Unscramble the key terms below and write the term inside the cells, by using the definitions shown.

esionl

- - - - - - - - - - - - - - - - -   is any mark on the skin that is not a normal part of the skin.

uelscam

- - - - - - - - - - - - - - - - -   are flat (nonelevated) marks on the skin where there is only a change in the normal
skin color.

athcesp

- - - - - - - - - - - - - - - - -   are large macules that are larger than 1 centimeter.

paupels

- - - - - - - - - - - - - - - - -   are raised areas on the skin that are generally smaller than 1 centimeter.

alqeusp

- - - - - - - - - - - - - - - - -   are papules that are larger than 1 centimeter.

duelson

- - - - - - - - - - - - - - - - -   are raised lesions that are larger and deeper in the skin. A nodule looks like a lump, but the skin can be
moved over the lesion.

ormust

- - - - - - - - - - - - - - - - -   are very large nodules.

sutuelp

- - - - - - - - - - - - - - - - -   is a clump of white blood cells that have formed and risen to the surface of the skin.

abcesesss

- - - - - - - - - - - - - - - - -   are extremely deep infections with pockets of pus.

silceev

- - - - - - - - - - - - - - - - -   is the medical term for blister.

lalub

- - - - - - - - - - - - - - - - -   is a large vesicle.

eahlw

- - - - - - - - - - - - - - - - -   is a raised red lesion associated with sensitivity or allergy; also called hives.

xocritaonise

- - - - - - - - - - - - - - - - -   are scratches on the skin.

reyhtema

- - - - - - - - - - - - - - - - -   refers to any area of redness associated with a lesion.

matemosah

- - - - - - - - - - - - - - - - -   are bruises.

raupurp

- - - - - - - - - - - - - - - - -   are hemorrhages of the blood vessels.

perorthpyhy

- - - - - - - - - - - - - - - - -   is thickening of a tissue.

ertaosisk

- - - - - - - - - - - - - - - - -   is a general term meaning thickening of the stratum corneum.

zemtiaztainoce

- - - - - - - - - - - - - - - - - -   refers to a combination of symptoms, including erythema, weeping, crusting, and present vesicles.

ntigniesel

- - - - - - - - - - - - - - - - - -   are freckles.

hroismascsyd

- - - - - - - - - - - - - - - - - -   are skin color abnormalities.

igmentopphyionat

- - - - - - - - - - - - - - - - - -   refers to any area with less than the normal amount of pigment.

petgoimi

- - - - - - - - - - - - - - - - - -   is a skin infection characterized by large, open, weeping lesions.

rnucleuf

- - - - - - - - - - - - - - - - - -   is a severe infection of the hair follicle. It is also known as a boil.

buncselrac

- - - - - - - - - - - - - - - - - -   are large boils that often result in abscesses.

Word Puzzle

Just like recognizing common skin conditions and the medications that may be prescribed to treat certain conditions, it is important to first be able to recognize the different terms that refer to different skin conditions. See if you can find terms related to skin conditions and treatment in the following word search. (*Hint:* the terms are also used in the word scramble above.)

```
F F D G T G H I N P A P W V E S I C L E L E S S S
K K W G Q G H I B P R P U L X S N O M U E E S M S
T W W E D H N I Q P A P U W C L K O U K L E T S L
R F G G T O G I G P G P G L O S N W D U L W U T S
P U S T U L E I S P A P U E R Y T H E M A E M S W
H R G G T B H I F P H H H S I E N E G N L W O K S
G U H H T B Q I G P A Y C L A S W A D M L Q R S W
B N H E T V S I H P A P U R T E P L A Q U E S T S
G C G J T Q M A C U L E S L I S W R F G G E S E X
W L T H L A S I F P A R X T O T N O D U L V S S S
Q E C Z E M A T I Z A T I O N S B V B G T V L S W
D T A T N V B I G P G R W G S S N O D B L E E W S
K E R A T O S I S P A O F L E S N O D U L E S Q W
F T B A I B C B H P A P U L E S B R D L L E I V S
G G U E G N E B H E A H U L E S N N D L E R O S S
T G N A I C S N V P D Y S C H R O M I A S E N X E
Y H C R N B S B B M A P W L E S H O M U L R S S P
Q H L A E N E N W P G P C G E S N E P U R P U R A
S B E T S W S Q Q T A P U G E S F T E U E R S V T
G G S A T Q S S S P H P W B H E M A T O M A S W C
E E R A R C S W V E B P U B F S G O I E L E S H H
F G R A T V S D V Z A P W N E S N G G U F R S W E
K G R A H Y P O P I G M E N T A T I O N L E S S S
```

CHAPTER 8

Essential Knowledge of Chemistry

Multiple Choice

Circle the correct answer.

1. An element is
   A. anything that takes up space and has substance.
   B. a chemical in its simplest form.
   C. the center of the atom.
   D. the smallest measurable amount of matter.

2. Matter is
   A. made up of carbon, oxygen, nitrogen, hydrogen, and sulfur.
   B. the bond between two amino acid groups.
   C. anything that takes up space and has substance.
   D. a catalyst.

3. An atom is the smallest
   A. measurable unit of an element.
   B. electron.
   C. measurable unit of a nucleus.
   D. electron that is negatively charged.

4. A substance that helps to cause a reaction, or speed up a reaction, without its atoms becoming a direct part of the reaction's products is called
   A. a distillation.
   B. a protein.
   C. a catalyst.
   D. a neutron.

5. A reaction between two elements or two compounds that results in chemical changes is called
   A. reactivity.
   B. a chemical change.
   C. chemical bonding.
   D. a chemical reaction.

6. Heating to remove one chemical from another is
   A. distillation.
   B. disintegration.
   C. biochemistry.
   D. ionic bonding.

7. The bond between two amino acid groups is called
   A. bonding.
   B. a peptide bond.
   C. chemical bonding.
   D. a chemical peptide.

8. A molecule is
   A. atoms and electrons.
   B. two or more atoms joined together.
   C. two or more ions joined together.
   D. charged atoms.

9. Protons are
   A. very small negatively charged particles within the atom.
   B. very large negatively charged particles within the atom.
   C. very small positively charged particles within the atom.
   D. made up of neutrons that are highly charged.

10. When atoms "steal" or "give away" electrons to each other, the resulting atoms with new charges are called
    A. ions.
    B. neutrons.
    C. protons.
    D. valences.

True/False

Mark T for true and F for false in the space provided.

1. ____ Electrons, which orbit the nucleus, are positively charged.

2. ____ The nucleus is positive because it is made up of positive protons and neutrons that have no charge.

3. ____ Atoms of the same element are exactly alike—they are the same size and weight and have the same number of protons.

4. ____ A compound is produced when molecules of two different elements join.

5. ____ A solution is a mixture of solvents.

6. ____ A mixture is produced when different elements or compounds are mixed together physically.

7. ____ A solute is the liquid part of the solution.

8. ____ pH refers to the measurement of hydrogen ions of a substance.

9. ____ The higher the pH of a substance, the more acidic it is; the lower the pH, the more alkaline the substance.

10. ____ A high pH increases the permeability of the skin, making it easier for bacteria, microorganisms, and other harmful substances to enter the body.

11. ____ Bases have a low concentration of hydrogen atoms and high pH values.

12. ____ Biochemistry is the study of chemicals and chemical reactions in the body.

13. ____ A polypeptide is a chain of polymers.

14. ____ Heat is one condition required for some chemical reactions.

15. ____ Most of the chemical reactions within the body are called organic reactions.

Fill in the Blank

Using the word bank below, fill in the blank to complete the sentence. The same word may be used more than once.

Word Bank

polymers	polysaccharides	pH	acidic	homogenous
amino acid	sulfur	alpha hydroxy	solution	ionization
saccharides	protein	acids (AHAs)	enzyme	poly
disaccharide	peptide bond	beta hydroxy	suspension	aldehyde
		acids (BHAs)	saturated	di

1. _____ can refer to any carbohydrate group.

2. The bond between two amino acid groups is called _____ ____.

3. A substance that is made up of carbon, oxygen, hydrogen, and ____ is called _____.

4. _____ means two saccharides are bonded together.

5. Many saccharides bonded together are called _____.

6. _____ ____ is the basic unit of a protein molecule.

7. Chains of carbon–carbon and carbon–hydrogen bonded together are called _____.

8. __ means two.

9. _____ can mean that a solution has absorbed as much solute as possible or that a molecule has taken on as many hydrogen atoms as it can.

10. The prefix ____ means many.

11. A proteolytic protein that is involved as a catalyst in chemical reactions such as those used to break down substances is called an _____.

12. The use of _____ _____ ____ _____ and ___ _____ ____ _____ in chemical peeling procedures is very important to the esthetician. The lower the ___, the more _____ the product is. When the ___ is lower than 3.0, the irritation potential of these exfoliation treatments increases.

13. A liquid solution in which the internal and external phases do not stay mixed for any length of time is called a _____. A _____ is usually not _____, therefore the mixture is not even throughout.

14. A _____ is a mixture of chemicals.

15. When a substance has been charged by changing atoms to ions the process is called _____.

16. An _____ is a compound with carbon and hydrogen, with a carbon, hydrogen, and oxygen group on the end of the molecule.

Define

Use the space provided to define these terms.

1. Element

_____

_____

_____

2. Electrons

_____

_____

_____

3. Covalent bond

_____

_____

_____

4. Solution

_____

_____

_____

5. pH

_____

_____

_____

_____

6. Chemical reactions

_____

_____

_____

7. Why is pH important to the esthetician?

_____

_____

_____

_____

_____

Word Scramble

Unscramble the key terms below and write the term inside the cells, by using the definitions shown.

emtelen

- - - - - - - - - - - - - - - - -   is a chemical in its simplest form.

tatrem

- - - - - - - - - - - - - - - - -   is anything that takes up space and has substance.

omta

- - - - - - - - - - - - - - - - -   is the smallest measurable unit of an element.

ucluesn

- - - - - - - - - - - - - - - - -   of the cell is made up largely of protein and is also responsible for building certain proteins.

trosncele

- - - - - - - - - - - - - - - - -   are negatively charged particles that orbit the nucleus of an atom. The exchange of these particles causes chemical reactions.

ontrosp

- - - - - - - - - - - - - - - - -   are very small, positively charged particles within the atom.

utonrsen

- - - - - - - - - - - - - - - - -   are very small, uncharged particles within the atom.

nosi

- - - - - - - - - - - - - - - - -   or charged atoms, are the resulting atoms with new charges when atoms "steal" or "give away" electrons to each other.

leucleom

- - - - - - - - - - - - - - - - -   is two or more atoms joined together.

lecenva

- - - - - - - - - - - - - - - - -   is the number of electrons in the outer energy level of an atom.

mponudoc

- - - - - - - - - - - - - - - - -   is produced when molecules of two different elements join.

ixurtem

- - - - - - - - - - - - - - - - -   is produced when different elements or compounds are mixed together physically.

oluitons

-------------------- is a mixture of chemicals.

nevtlos

-------------------- is the liquid part of a solution.

luetso

-------------------- is the solid part of a solution.

qutaoine

-------------------- describe a chemical reaction such that equal numbers of the same atom are on either side of the reaction.

ochibeismtry

-------------------- is the study of chemicals and chemical reactions within the body.

ymerslop

-------------------- are chains of carbon–carbon and carbon–hydrogen bonded together.

rointep

-------------------- is made of carbon, oxygen, nitrogen, hydrogen, and sulfur.

tidpeep

-------------------- is a chain of amino acids.

ylopepidetp

-------------------- is a chain of amino acid molecules (peptides).

hiaredccas

-------------------- can refer to any carbohydrate group.

accaridehosonm

-------------------- is one saccharide by itself.

accridehasid

-------------------- means two saccharides are bonded together.

saccaridehylop

-------------------- means many saccharides are bonded together.

sesba

-------------------- have a low concentration of hydrogen atoms and high pH values.

Word Puzzle

The chemical components of any type of matter are often too small to be seen with the naked eye, but under a strong microscope chemical reactions and chemical components such as molecules can be seen. See if you can find chemistry terms in the following word search. (*Hint*: the terms are also used in the word scramble above.)

```
A O D Y S A C M O N O S A C C H A R I D E E H N
P W I Y D G H I H A R I D E S T O P R O T W J W
B O S W S A C X Q W R I R R E T W P R O T E I F
P Q A Y E P W T H A P I D E L E C T R O N S G N
C F C E S O L U T I O N W Q H T O P R O H E I E
P V C Y H L J R D A L G D U S T E P R Q T Q W G
E B H H E Y C E H Q Y I B A S E S P R O W E I D
P O A Y Q P K C F A M G D T H T F P S W T E W F
G Q R W S E C C H D E I Q I S T Q P O O W W S E
P O I Y T P L C F P R O T O N S O P L G B E I F
J W D W S T C C H A S I D N S O W P U G I S I G
P P E P T I D E H A R I R E S L O P T O O E F H
E O L Y E D M C W I G I E E F V A L E N C E I N
P R L E S E C C M O L E C U L E G P R T H E G E
K O L Y R A C C H N G G O E S N O P R G E W I L
P F L N U C L E U S R I M E A T O M G O M E G E
L O L Y S A M C Q H R G P E T F O P Q Q I W I M
P R L Y W F C N E U T R O N S T O P R T S E J E
Q Y L Y S A M C H H D H U E H W G P R O T E I N
P O L F H G C N S M R I N E S T N P R F R F K T
P O L Y S A C C H A R I D E F E O P G O Y E L H
W F L Y G A C C H T H H D E S T G P R G T G I N
P O L G S F M K W T R I F E K H O P N B T E N G
S A C C H A R I D E G I B E S T T P Q T T G I J
P O L Y S A C L H R R E D E J W O P R O T E O N
```

CHAPTER 9

Cosmetic Chemistry and Functional Ingredients

Multiple Choice

Circle the correct answer.

1. Functional ingredients make up the main part of any cosmetic or skin-care product by
   A. causing changes in the physical appearance of the skin.
   B. being active ingredients.
   C. helping the product to spread across the skin, keeping the product mixed and uniform in texture, adjusting the pH of a product, and keeping the product fresh.
   D. thickening products with performance ingredients.

2. The largest category of functional ingredients is
   A. performance ingredients.
   B. active ingredients.
   C. performance agents.
   D. vehicles.

3. Performance ingredients are
   A. ingredients that cause actual physical changes to the appearance of the skin.
   B. functional agents.
   C. vehicles.
   D. functional ingredients that help promote actual physical changes to the appearance of the skin.

4. The terms "active agent" or "active ingredients" imply that the substance is a
   A. drug.   B. vehicle.   C. performance ingredient.   D. functional ingredient.

5. The most common vehicle ingredient is
   A. oil.   B. wax.   C. water.   D. silicone.

6. Deionizing water means
   A. the water has had minerals and other trace elements removed from it.
   B. the process neutralizes ions that can cross-react with other ingredients or make the product unstable.
   C. the process makes it an excellent spreading agent.
   D. it is attracted to and binds to humectants used in moisturizers.

7. Ingredients that lubricate the skin; work as vehicles to help spread other performance ingredients; and give cosmetics a soft, smooth feeling are
   A. oils.   B. polymers.   C. emollients.   D. lubricators.

8. Chemists often refer to chemicals that stop water evaporation from the skin as
   A. protectants.   B. emollients.   C. petroleum.   D. barriers.

9. Silicones are used in skin-care products because
   A. they are excellent exfoliants.

   B. they are biologically inert, meaning they are unlikely to cause allergic reactions.

   C. of the delivery system.

   D. they are derived from natural sources.

10. Polymers are synthetic molecular structures that
    A. are spreading agents that help many ingredients adhere to the skin surface or penetrate performance ingredients.

    B. are used in products as an anti-inflammatory.

    C. are state-of-the-art spreading agents that can cause irritation.

    D. are spreading agents that are a blend of fatty acids.

True/False

Write T for true and F for false in the space provided.

1. ____ Fatty acids are made of a synthetic substance.

2. ____ Fatty acids help to give a soft, firm texture to lotions and creams and are good emollient lubricants.

3. ____ Although fatty acids such as myristic acid, palmitic acid, lauric acid, oleic acid, and stearic acid may have many good properties for cosmetic use, they can be comedogenic.

4. ____ Alcohols have a negative connotation in the cosmetic industry, and it is much undeserved.

5. ____ The term "alcohol" is a chemical term that means an oxygen atom and a hydrogen atom have attached themselves to the end of a carbon chain.

6. ____ Cetyl alcohol is used as a foam booster in detergent cleansers.

7. ____ Fatty esters feel very oily compared with other types of fatty ingredients.

8. ____ An ester is formed when an organic acid combines with an alcohol.

9. ____ The easiest way to identify a fatty ester in an ingredient label is that fatty esters have the suffix -ate.

10. ____ Fatty esters are both functional and performance ingredients that can be used to smooth the surface of the hair or skin; to serve as a protectant; and to help replace esters that are missing from older, dryer skin types.

11. ____ Fatty esters are never comedogenic.

12. ____ Isopropyl myristate, isopropyl palmitate, ethylhexyl palmitate, propylene glycol dicaprate/dicaprylate are all frequently used fatty esters in skin-care and cosmetic formulation.

Fill in the Blank

Using the word bank below, fill in the blank to complete the sentence. The same word may be used more than once.

Word Bank

surfactants	sodium lauryl sulfate	biologically inert	bacteria	emollient
anionic	disodium lauryl	petroleum	emulsifiers	cocamidopropyl
cationic	sulfosuccinate	fungi	rancid	betaine
amphoteric	shell	yeast	esters	silicone compounds
nonionic	cyclomethicone	protectants		

1. _____ cause a cosmetic to be able to slip across or onto the skin.

2. A cosmetic product that has discoloration and/or odor as a result of oxidization is _____.

3. Chemists often refer to chemicals that stop water evaporation as _____.

4. _____ form when an organic acid combines with an alcohol.

5. An ingredient that gives the skin lubrication and the product a soft, smooth feeling is an _____.

6. The four basic types of _____ are _____, _____, _____, and _____.

7. Three types of surfactant ingredients frequently used in cleansers are _____ _____ _____, _____ _____ _____, and _____ _____.

8. A ____ around very small droplets allows emulsifiers to remain suspended in a solution of water.

9. Three examples of silicones frequently used both as protectants and as spreading agents are _____, dimethicone, and phenyl trimethicone.

10. _____ keep water-and-oil solutions mixed well.

11. Two substances that are unlikely to produce allergic or irritant reactions and will not react with normal chemical reactions in the skin are _____ ____ _____ and _____ _____.

12. The three main types of microorganisms present in cosmetic formulations are ____, ____, and _____.

Matching

Match the term with the best description, and write the letter of the term in the space provided.

Description   *Terms*

1. ____ The oil droplets in an oil-in-water emulsion.   A. distilled

2. ____ Water that has had minerals and other trace   B. micelle
elements removed from it.

3. ____ Prevents urine and soggy diapers from irritating   C. chelating agent
a baby's sensitive skin.

4. ____ Water-loving.   D. silicone

5. ____ Adjusting the pH of a product to make it more   E. lipophilic
acceptable to the skin.

6. ____ The process by which oxygen is exposed to certain   F. buffering
ingredients, resulting in a breakdown of the ingredient.

7. ____ Fat-loving.   G. oil

8. ____ Over-emulsification of an ingredient.   H. petroleum

9. ____ Chemicals that are added to cosmetic formulas to   I. hydrophilic
prevent oxidation.

10. ____ Water-in-oil emulsion is primarily this solution.   J. globules

11. ____ A chemical that is added to cosmetics to improve   K. antioxidants
the efficiency of the preservative.

12. ____ An emollient that leaves a protective film on the   L. oxidation
surface of the skin.

Define

Use the space provided to define these terms.

1. Preservatives

_____

_____

_____

2. Antioxidants

_____

_____

_____

3. Buffering

_____

_____

_____

4. Microencapsulation

_____

_____

_____

5. Phospholipids

_____

_____

_____

6. Liposomes

_____

_____

_____

7. Loaded liposome

_____

_____

_____

8. Microsponge

_____

_____

9. Nanosphere

_____

_____

_____

Word Scramble

Unscramble the key terms below and write the term inside the cells, by using the definitions shown.

hiclesve

----------------- are ingredients used as spreading agents.

ionizignde

----------------- is the process of neutralizing ions in water that can cross-react in a product.

laltitinosid

----------------- is the process of purifying water.

olleitsnem

----------------- are somewhat like occlusives in that they mostly lie on the surface of the skin and prevent water loss. They also help "fill in the cracks" of dry, dehydrated skin.

tetanstcrop

----------------- are chemicals that stop water evaporation.

ertoaltmup

----------------- prevents urine and soggy diapers from irritating the baby's sensitive skin.

islionce

----------------- is an emollient that leaves a protective film on the surface of the skin.

clopneycsatloixean

----------------- is a silicone compound often used as a spreading agent.

ehticoenmid

----------------- is a smaller, lighter version of silicone.

clmeohienocyct

----------------- is a type of silicone used primarily as a vehicle or emollient.

lxneaioequsilsythempoyl

------------------- is another type of silicone-based vehicle.

xeasw

----------------- are thick, fatty substances that are derived primarily from plants and used as emollients in skin-care products.

scoitsyiv

----------------- is the thickness and liquidity of a solution, skin-care product, or cosmetic.

sterse

----------------- are modified fatty substances that are used primarily as vehicles and emollients in skin-care products and cosmetics.

tantcasfrus

----------------- are chemicals in cosmetics that enable the cosmetic to slip across or onto the skin.

genstreted

----------------- are surfactants used for cleansing.

siifrslume

----------------- are chemicals that keep water and oil solutions well mixed.

hilipcolip

----------------- means "fat-loving."

dropyhihlic

----------------- means "water-loving."

loulesbg

----------------- are oil droplets in an oil-in-water emulsion.

Word Puzzle

Just like being able to identify the different components and substances (or ingredients) in different products or compositions, it is important to recognize the different terminology and chemical compositions of products. See if you can find product-related terms in the following word search. (*Hint*: the terms are also used in the word scramble above.)

```
S Q W E A D T A N T D D I G I E R S H V C L E S E
W S C Q A W T A N B E S T E R S R P G I H L E W T
G D S M S V T Q B T T S D G B G G O G S C L F S E
L Q D N A N R A N W E W I F I H G L H C F E E W E
O U Q E F E T W E T R S S S W W R Y E O C M E S R
B Q A W A F E A N W G S L F B E F M H S C O R F E
U U C D E B T A G T E W I F I S V E H I C L E S E
L G W V A C G A N D N S P D D E T T E T F L E I E
E U Q G E C T W N T T S O F I Q R H H Y C I R L Q
S U R F A C T A N T S Q P F S E T Y J I C E E I E
S U R F A C D X N W S S H D T W R L H H E N W C W
S D C S E F G E M U L S I F I E R S J I C T E O E
F U Y V D B T S N Q S S L F L E T I H I N S E N Q
S W C F A C V A N T S W I D L E E L H F C L E E E
D U L B F F T P R O T E C T A N T S G I N L G T W
S W O W A N D A N S S Q I F T G H E H T C L E S E
G U M F G H Y D R O P H I L I C R Q N I V L E R E
S U E Q A E H A N T S F I D O E G U H W C L W S Q
V U T F J C D E I O N I Z I N G R I J I S L E H E
S S H W A F T A N D S W I V I F G O H Q C L W S N
S U I F K C T A N T S F I F N E R X J I R L E F E
B U C Y C L O P E N T A S I L O X A N E C L X S W
S U O G A C D A N V S S I S B E G N H E F L E W E
N U N F G C T A N T S Q I F D I M E T H I C O N E
S P E T R O L A T U M S I F I E R S H I C L E S E
```

CHAPTER 10

Performance Ingredients and Active Ingredients

Multiple Choice

Circle the correct answer.

1. The FDA defines a drug as
   A. an article intended to be rubbed, poured, sprinkled, or otherwise applied to the human body or any part thereof for cleansing, beautifying, promoting physical attractiveness, or altering the appearance.
   B. a performance agent that alters the appearance of the skin.
   C. an active ingredient that affects the appearance of the skin structure.
   D. an article (other than food) intended to affect the structure of any function of the body.

2. Ingredients within a skin-care product or cosmetic that actually change the appearance of the skin are known as
   A. performance agents.
   B. drugs.
   C. vehicles.
   D. performance ingredients.

3. Active ingredients are substances within a drug intended to cause
   A. appearance changes.
   B. structural or biochemical functional change.
   C. appearance and chemical changes.
   D. chemical changes.

4. Performance ingredients are intended to cause
   A. reparative changes.
   B. biochemical function changes.
   C. structural changes.
   D. appearance changes.

5. An example of a performance ingredient is
   A. an emulsifier.
   B. an oil-in-water solution.
   C. an emollient.
   D. a water-in-oil solution.

6. Cosmeceutical ingredients are found in skin-care products that are
   A. drugs meant to treat diseases.
   B. skin health promoting and have positive effects on the skin.
   C. performance agents that have been recognized by the FDA.
   D. skin health promoting and change the structural biochemistry of the skin.

7. Cleansing agents are of
   A. two types.
   B. three types.
   C. four types.
   D. one basic type.

8. Types of cleansers may be detergents or
   A. emollients.
   B. emulsions.
   C. vehicles.
   D. soaps.

9. An active ingredient that makes a cleanser foam is a
   A. detergent.
   B. soap.
   C. salt.
   D. superfatted ingredient.

10. A defatting agent is a detergent that
    A. acts as a vehicle. B. acts as a cleanser. C. removes fats and lipids. D. is a foaming agent.

11. Soap is a defatting product made up of
    A. salts of fatty acids. B. fatty acids. C. oils. D. fats.

12. Superfatted soaps are used for
    A. extremely oily skin. B. acne. C. fragile, dry, dehydrated skin. D. combination skin.

13. Fatty additives in soap often start with the word
    A. fatty. B. sodium. C. ester. D. stearic.

14. Cleansing milks are called
    A. emollient cleansers. B. detergent cleansers. C. emulsion cleansers. D. foaming cream-type cleansers.

15. Emulsion cleansers should always be followed by
    A. a moisturizer. B. a hydrator. C. a protectant. D. a toner.

True/False

Write T for true and F for false in the space provided.

1. ____ One advantage of a cleansing milk is that it is good for sensitive skin.

2. ____ The primary function of a toner is to exfoliate the skin.

3. ____ Astringents have a tightening effect on the skin or pore appearance.

4. ____ Witch hazel is a strong astringent.

5. ____ Isopropyl alcohol is a strong drying alcohol used as a cleansing agent to remove excess oil from very oily skin.

6. ____ Sodium PCA is an antibacterial and keratolytic agent.

7. ____ NMFs (natural moisturizing factors) are hydrating agents found within the cells and within the intercellular cement.

8. ____ Lipid replacement is accomplished by applying a specialized group of lipids to the skin.

9. ____ Some well-known ingredients that contain lipids are linoleic acid, evening primrose oil, borage oil, and soy sterols.

10. ____ Lipids alone are effective for hydration.

11. ____ Hydrophilic ingredients, or humectants, are oil loving.

12. ____ Sodium PCA is an excellent hydrator.

13. ____ Glycerin is a strong water binder; however, if used alone over time it can make the skin drier.

14. ____ Propylene glycol can increase permeability of the skin, and in doing so can also cause problems for sensitive or dry skin with impaired barrier function.

15. ____ Hyaluronic acid can hold up to 400 times its own weight in water.

Fill in the Blank

Using the word bank below, fill in the blank to complete the sentence. The same word or phrase may be used more than once.

Word Bank

hyaluronic acid	emollients	emulsions	malic acid	sebaceous secretions
collagen	alipidic	proteases	tartaric acid	dehydrated
elastin	400 times	alpha hydroxy acids	broad-spectrum	glycolic acid
substantives	reactive oxygen	(AHAs)	contraindications	barrier functions
mucopolysaccharides	species	beta hydroxy acid	exfoliation	improvement
occlusives	antioxidants	(BHA)	inflammation cascade	
petroleum	water-in-oil			

1. _____ is known as sodium hyaluronate and can hold up to _____ its own weight in water.

2. Carbohydrate–lipid complexes called _____ are good water binders and are considered to be a "mother molecule" to hyaluronic acid.

3. _____ and _____ are large long-chain proteins that help to bind water to the skin and prevent water loss.

4. Ingredients that attach themselves well to the surface of the skin, spreading out to protect and hydrate the skin, are called _____.

5. Heavy, large molecules that sit on top of the skin preventing moisture loss are called _____.

6. One example of an occlusive is _____. Although it can be helpful in keeping foreign bodies out of the skin, it can cause a backup of _____ _____.

7. _____ are similar to occlusives in that they lie on the surface of the skin to prevent water loss and help to "fill in the cracks" of _____ skin.

8. A lack of lipids, or _____, means that this skin type does not produce enough lipids to keep the skin moist. _____ emulsions are designed for this type of skin.

9. ____ _____ ____ _____ make up a family of naturally occurring mild acids; two lesser known of them are ____ ___ and _____ ___, and the one that is the most well known is called _____ ___.

10. ___ _____ ___ _____ is known for _____, which is the removal of dead skin cells from the surface of the skin by loosening the bond between dead corneum cells and dissolving part of the surface intercellular cement that holds the epidermal cells together.

11. A _____ sunscreen with an SPF (sun protection factor) of at least 15 is necessary when using alpha hydroxy acids or beta hydroxy acids.

12. New information now indicates that routine use of alpha hydroxy acids improves _____ _____ of the epidermis; and long-term studies show an _____ of collagen content in the dermis.

13. Pregnant or nursing women, clients taking Accutane®, and clients who have had a recent laser resurfacing procedure are just a few of the clients who have _____ for the use of alpha hydroxy acids and beta hydroxy acids.

14. The _____ _____ is a series of biochemical reactions that lead to the production of self-destruct enzymes in the skin called _____. This process causes destruction of _____ and _____ fibers necessary for firm, smooth skin.

15. Many scientists believe that free radicals, or reactive _____ _____, are responsible for aging the skin and the body. To combat some of the damage, _____ can neutralize free radicals before they attack cell membranes at the beginning of the _____ _____.

Short Answer

1. _____, _____, and _____ are three self-destruct enzymes that cause destruction of collagen, elastin, and hyaluronic acid in the skin.

2. The routine use of topical antioxidants can help to improve the _____ signs of aging.

3. When different types of antioxidants are combined in a formulation, the formulation is said to be a _____ _____.

4. The invention of liposomes and microencapsulation provides a way to keep the reactive substances in antioxidants _____ until they can be used. The processes also help to keep the antioxidants _____ to be used as a performance agent on the skin.

5. _____ _____, _____, and _____ ____ are common antioxidant ingredients used in skin-care products today.

6. _____ is a newly discovered powerful antioxidant.

7. _____ are a recent discovery in the use of amino acids for aging skin in the treatment of wrinkles and lack of elasticity.

8. The most often used peptide ingredient is _____ _____. It is also known as _____.

9. _____ is a peptide ingredient that is used in wrinkle-relaxing creams.

10. Retinol is a natural form of _____ that seems to stimulate cell repair and regulate skin functions and is theorized to be necessary to stimulate collagen production.

11. Results from anti-aging ingredients are best when used in a combination including a _____, _____, and a _____ serum along with ____ _____ ___ or ___ _____ ___ gels or creams.

12. Many plant extracts are often used for their _____ properties.

13. Plant extracts are natural complexes of various _____. There can be literally _____ of chemicals that make up a single plant extract.

14. Many ingredients can influence or worsen redness-prone or _____ ___.

15. Ingredients such as sphingolipids, glycosphingolipids, phospholipids, cholesterol, and certain fatty acids are all ____ _____ _____ that can serve as a complex patch and reinforce barrier function in sensitive skin.

16. Many antioxidants may serve as _____ _____ by interfering with the _____ _____ that can lead to redness.

17. ____ ___ _____, stearyl glycyrrhetinate, and zinc oxide are all ingredients known for their soothing benefits.

18. OTC drugs are required by law to use special chart labels called _____ _____ to inform the consumer of what the product is used for, how to use the product, and possible side effects and contraindications.

19. _____ _____ will always be listed first along with the purpose of the ingredient.

20. The two types of sunscreen ingredients are _____ ___ _____.

21. Two ingredients seen in physical sunscreens are ___ _____ and _____ _____.

Define/Describe the Following Ingredients

1. Benzoyl peroxide

   _____

   _____

   _____

   _____

2. Salicylic acid

   _____

   _____

   _____

   _____

3. Hydroquinone

   _____

   _____

   _____

   _____

4. Kojic acid

   _____

   _____

   _____

   _____

5. Glycolic acid

   _____

   _____

   _____

   _____

6. Sulfur

   _____

   _____

   _____

   _____

7. Papain

   _____

   _____

   _____

   _____

Word Scramble

Unscramble the key terms below and write the term inside the cells, by using the definitions shown.

ticsmsoce

- - - - - - - - - - - - - - - - - -   are articles intended to be applied to the human body to alter the appearance or promote attractiveness.

smceeuitalscco

- - - - - - - - - - - - - - - - - -   are products that are not drugs intended to treat disease, but they still benefit the skin in a positive way.

tergnetsde

- - - - - - - - - - - - - - - - - -   are cleansing ingredients that help break up and remove fatty residues and other impurities from the skin.

erfattdepus

- - - - - - - - - - - - - - - - - -   cleansing agents that have had fat added.

mecttanuh

- - - - - - - - - - - - - - - - - -   is an ingredient that attracts water.

bitlorso

- - - - - - - - - - - - - - - - - -   is a humectant.

zuleena

- - - - - - - - - - - - - - - - - -   is a hydrocarbon that is derived from the chamomile flower.

hamoimelc

- - - - - - - - - - - - - - - - - -   is a soothing agent.

ablolosbi

- - - - - - - - - - - - - - - - - -   is a soothing agent that is added to cosmetics designed for sensitive skin.

gopilisnisph

- - - - - - - - - - - - - - - - - -   are lipid materials that are a natural part of the intercellular cement.

goliidspinsphcoylg

- - - - - - - - - - - - - - - - - -   are lipid materials that are a natural part of the intercellular cement.

misedarce

- - - - - - - - - - - - - - - - - -   are lipid materials that are a natural part of the intercellular cement.

phopilisdsoph

- - - - - - - - - - - - - - - - - -   are naturally moisturizing humectants found within the skin.

yercollg

- - - - - - - - - - - - - - - - - -   is a humectant that is a natural part of the intercellular cement.

uaenlasq

- - - - - - - - - - - - - - - - - -   is a lipid material that is a natural part of the intercellular cement.

oeslterloch

- - - - - - - - - - - - - - - - - -   is a lipid material that is a natural part of the intercellular cement.

ycrinegl

- - - - - - - - - - - - - - - - - -   is a humectant and is a very strong water binder.

cchairdessaolypocum

- - - - - - - - - - - - - - - - -   are carbohydrate–lipid complexes that are also good water binders.

gaenlolc

- - - - - - - - - - - - - - - - -   is a large, long-chain molecular protein that lies on top of the skin and binds water; it also helps prevent water loss.

saintel

- - - - - - - - - - - - - - - - -   is a large, long-chain molecular protein that lies on top of the skin and binds water; it also helps prevent water loss.

tantivesssub

- - - - - - - - - - - - - - - - -   are ingredients that attach themselves well to the surface of the skin, sort of spreading out across the skin, to protect and hydrate the surface.

lsivesucco

- - - - - - - - - - - - - - - - -   are heavy, large molecules that sit on top of the skin and prevent moisture loss.

oltumarpet

- - - - - - - - - - - - - - - - -   prevents urine and soggy diapers from irritating the baby's sensitive skin.

ollentsime

- - - - - - - - - - - - - - - - -   are somewhat like occlusives in that they mostly lie on the surface of the skin and prevent water loss. They also help "fill in the cracks" of dry, dehydrated skin.

lidipica

- - - - - - - - - - - - - - - - -   means "lack of lipids." These skin types do not produce enough lipids.

Word Puzzle

Looking for specific ingredients and knowing what these ingredients do for the skin is important. See if you can find terms related to performance ingredients and active ingredients in the following word search. (*Hint*: the terms are also used in the word scramble above.)

```
R C R W E G L Y C O S P H I N G O L I P I D S Q
G W U C B G K Y C O S P F Q H G O E I J I D U S
J C S E E G L W Y O W G H I B G O L W P U F P P
W Q U R A M U C O P O L Y S A C C H A R I D E S
C C T A W G H H C O W Y W H G R O G H K I W R D
V H U M E C T A N T S C F I G G H L I P J D F S
C O U I N G L M Q O E E Q F E G O E I O E W A W
F L W D E G J O C S O R B I T O L L W C I D T S
C E U E M G L M K O S O H I W G N W I C Q S T Q
E S X S E E H I C O G L Y C E R I N I L I D E S
C T U V L P L L M O H G W W L G O L W U D Q D D
T E Y V K H D E C O S P H I A S W L I S I P Y A
C R U B E O W Y N B Q S U B S T A N T I V E S B
Y O Z A U S V D C I S P W E T G K W I V W T W S
X L U C E P A Y H S W W A I I E O L E E I R S D
C K F C F H Q J C A Z U L E N E E E I S G O D E
Z L C W E O W Y Q B S P I W J K O L E P I L S T
P N O C W L F K C O S P P I K G S Q U A L A N E
O E S P H I N G O L I P I D S F M L F P I T E R
C V M W E P Q Y C O S E D I N G O F I B W U S G
D Q E C F I L Q E L G P I H W B M L W P I M A E
C C T S E D W Y N O S D C O L L A G E N S D S N
W S I C W S R N C O E P W I N G O L I W I D E T
C C C Q E G E Y R O S W H B E M O L L I E N T S
C O S M E C E U T I C A L S D G N L W P I D S S
```

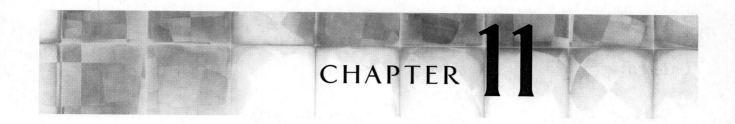

CHAPTER 11

Skin Care Products

Multiple Choice

Circle the correct answer.

1. The two most important factors in recommending skin-care products are
   A. the esthetician's own experiences with a product and personal knowledge.
   B. extensive research and attending product orientations.
   C. the esthetician's education and knowledge of skin analysis.
   D. having a good relationship with your sales representative and staying on top of the trends.

2. The two primary types of cleansers are
   A. rinsable detergent and milk types.
   B. clear gels and milky creams.
   C. lotion types and detergent gels.
   D. detergent and soap.

3. The ingredient disodium lauryl sulfosuccinate is
   A. a product ingredient for dry skin.
   B. a product ingredient for oily and combination skin.
   C. a product ingredient for super-sensitive dry skin.
   D. a surfactant ingredient for use in foaming cleansers that can be used on more than one skin type.

4. When sodium lauryl sulfate is listed lower in the product ingredient list, it means
   A. it is a strong ingredient meant for oily skin types.
   B. it is not nearly as concentrated as if it were listed first.
   C. it contains emollient ingredients.
   D. it is an ingredient for a gel cleanser.

5. Benzoyl peroxide usually is used for
   A. sensitive skin.   B. dry, acne-prone skin.   C. oily, acne-prone skin.   D. thin skin, as an exfoliant.

6. A milk cleanser should be used by a client with
   A. acne and oily skin.
   B. drier skin or as a first step for combination skin.
   C. oily skin.
   D. older skin.

7. Toners for oily skin act as
   A. an astringent.   B. an emollient.   C. an emulsifier.   D. a product for tightening.

8. A toner for normal skin may contain
   A. benzoyl peroxide.   B. allantoin.   C. sulfur.   D. an astringent.

9. The biggest skin health benefit that can be contained in a product for day use is
   A. a sunscreen.   B. an exfoliant.   C. an AHA.   D. a moisturizer.

10. Sodium hyaluronate, glycerin, and butylene glycol act as
    A. exfoliants.   B. emollients.   C. hydrating agents.   D. emulsifiers.

11. Alipidic (oil-dry), dehydrated, mature skin is best supported by the use of
    A. a cream.   B. a gel.   C. a lotion.   D. water.

12. Squalane is an ingredient intended for use by a client with
    A. skin that tends to plug easily.
    B. skin that does not tend to develop comedones.
    C. skin that is oily.
    D. skin that is thicker.

True/False

Write T for true and F for false in the space provided.

1. ____ Ampoules are sealed vials of concentrated ingredients designed to give ultra-intensive treatment to the skin.

2. ____ Ampoules have often been replaced by serums in the United States.

3. ____ Serums contain ingredients that are often placed in liposomes and use other advanced delivery systems that may contain antioxidants, peptides, and lipids.

4. ____ Firming serums are often used for younger, oily, acne-prone skin.

5. ____ Anhydrous means that the skin is sensitive.

6. ____ Serums that contain a specific lipid complex are intended to mimic the proportions of lipids found naturally in the normal barrier function of skin.

7. ____ Alpha hydroxy acid formulations work to exfoliate dead skin cells and are excellent as sunscreen ingredients.

8. ____ Alpha hydroxy acids are usually in a gel form.

9. ____ Hydroquinone is an excellent melanocyte suppressant for sensitive skin.

10. ____ Benzoyl peroxide is designed for acneic skin, grades I and II, and both teenagers and adults can use this active ingredient to exfoliate debris from the follicle.

Short Answer

1. Day creams should have a _____ for optimum benefit.

2. A protection product intended for oily and combination skin for day should be _____.

3. It is illegal to claim sunscreen protection and not list the _____ _____ on a drug facts label.

4. Day creams almost always contain either an _____ or _____ ingredient that helps hold moisture in the surface layers of the skin.

5. Products used for day should have an SPF (sun protection factor) of at least __ to shield against routine UVA-UVB exposure during daily activities.

6. Night creams are often _____ than day creams and contain more _____ ingredients.

7. Ingredients such as *Aloe barbadensis* gel, *Matricaria* extract, and green tea extract are often used in products for _____ skin.

8. "Fragrance-free" and "dermatologist-tested" should be included on the label of a product intended for _____ ___.

9. Oily-combination, dehydrated skin may break out easily and needs products containing ingredients that are _____ and may contain ingredients that are mostly _____.

10. Salicylic acid (beta hydroxy acid) is an excellent ingredient for night treatment for ___ _____ ___.

Define and Describe Function

1. Cleanser

_____

_____

_____

_____

_____

_____

_____

2. Toner

_____

_____

_____

_____

_____

_____

3. Cream

_____

_____

_____

_____

_____

_____

4. Gel

_____

_____

_____

_____

_____

_____

5. Mask

_____

_____

_____

_____

_____

_____

6. Skin lightener

_____

_____

_____

_____

_____

_____

7. Exfoliant

_____

_____

_____

_____

_____

_____

8. List the seven basic steps in developing new skin-care products:

A. _____

B. _____

C. _____

D. _____

E. _____

F. _____

G. _____

Word Scramble

Unscramble the key terms below and write the term inside the cells, by using the definitions shown.

ownrgni riah

- - - - - - - - - - - - - - -   is an infected follicle caused by a hair that grows into the side of the follicle wall.

mpoulesa

- - - - - - - - - - - - - - -   are sealed vials of concentrated ingredients designed to give intensive treatment to a skin condition.

erumss

- - - - - - - - - - - - - - -   are products containing concentrated ingredients that are usually in pump or tincture bottles.

nhyroudsar

- - - - - - - - - - - - - - -   means that a product does not contain water.

yee eamscr

- - - - - - - - - - - - - - -   are designed for the skin around the eye area.

cekn mearcs

- - - - - - - - - - - - - - -   are made with more emollients and less humectant, because the neck area has thinner skin that dries easily.

saksm

- - - - - - - - - - - - - - -   are designed to treat a variety of skin problems, from oil-dryness to acne.

xfloinatse

- - - - - - - - - - - - - - -   usually come in the form of scrubs. They are water-based products containing a humectant mixed with some sort of abrasive agent such as almond meal or polyethylene granules.

totepyorp

- - - - - - - - - - - - - - -   is a product sample that has been developed by the chemist and is ready to be tried.

Word Puzzle

Using your powers of observation, see if you can find terms related to skin-care products in the following word search. (*Hint:* the terms are also used in the word scramble above.)

```
P G O T R E G Y P E D D X B H S Y P E
B R E A G Y T W W E C R F Q F Q M R E
K F T D X E A D G H A I V M S G M E X
P R N O K C O H Y M E N F A B E H K F
K F E D A R D G H A X G V S S G M E O
P R C T O E T D P R D R W K N A M Y L
D G K C Q A N H Y D R O U S A H M S I
L V C F G M R L Q G H W U H S D M Y A
S E R U M S A H S R S N H Y P O U S N
W E E T O D N O U S P H G H R R L Q T
O T A R S P R O K O H A M P O U L E S
R T M Y M O K Y C R T I S E T M O T E
Y C S F R W V E W E W R O H O E W E W
P R O H M Q I T Q Q K F T D T X B R E
G Y P E D D X B H S S G M E Y H S D M
P R O K O H Y M E F R T Y M P P R O H
P P E T D Y C R T P P E T D E C R T Y
```

CHAPTER 12

Claims in Cosmetics

Multiple Choice

Circle the correct answer.

1. The Food and Drug Administration (FDA)
   A. is the federal agency that approves cosmetics and drugs.

   C. approves cosmetics and food.

   B. passed the Food, Drug, and Cosmetic Act.

   D. is the federal agency designed to ensure safety of consumer products such as food, cosmetics, and drugs.

2. The FDA only regulates the cosmetic industry
   A. when the agency disapproves of a claim or product.

   C. when a company does not register its products.

   B. when a product becomes a drug.

   D. if the company of a product states "it improves the appearance."

3. The Food and Drug Act of 1938 defines cosmetics as
   A. articles intended to affect the structure or any function of the body.

   C. articles intended to be rubbed, poured, sprinkled, or otherwise applied to the human body or any part thereof for cleansing, beautifying, promoting attractiveness, or altering the appearance.

   B. an intention to affect the structure of the skin.

   D. articles that claim to cleanse, beautify, promote attractiveness, or alter the structure or function of the skin.

4. The difference between a cosmetic and a drug is
   A. a drug is intended to affect the structure and function of the body

   C. a cosmetic is intended to affect the structure and function of the body.

   B. a drug improves the skin's appearance.

   D. a cosmetic claims to affect the function of the skin.

5. Registering a product as a drug means
   A. the new ingredients have been approved.

   C. the product is safe for use by the public.

   B. that the product must have had substantial testing to support its ingredient claims, efficacy, and safety.

   D. that the company has filed for "new ingredient" testing.

6. Estheticians must
   A. state exactly what the product will do for a client.

   C. claim that a product will remove red capillaries if it is intended to do so.

   B. be careful about making claims about a cosmetic that is a drug claim.

   D. state the actual chemical reaction that occurs in products.

7. A proper way of describing the benefits of a product is as follows:
   A. "This eye cream will take down swelling in the eye area."
   B. "This product will stimulate circulation and remove puffiness around the eye area."
   C. "This eye cream will help to reduce the appearance of swelling in the eye area."
   D. "This eye cream will take away dark circles."

8. Cosmeceuticals are products
   A. that are designed for appearance improvement but may have positive physiological effects on the skin on a cellular level.
   B. that offer structural change of the skin.
   C. about which estheticians can legally explain the actual chemical reactions to their clients.
   D. that are really drugs.

9. The Federal Packaging and Labeling Act requires
   A. manufacturers to list ingredients on their products in order of priority.
   B. ingredients to be listed on the outermost packaging so that the consumer may easily find it.
   C. ingredients to be listed on the container, initially to protect consumers who suffered from allergic reactions to particular ingredients.
   D. the names of the chemicals to be listed by their trade names.

10. The ingredients on the label of a product
    A. must be listed in order of performance function.
    B. must be in order of ingredients that are less than 1 percent.
    C. must be in order of natural ingredients.
    D. must be in order of the concentration at which they are present in the product.

True/False

Write T for true and F for false in the space provided.

1. ____ In 1938 the Food, Drug and Cosmetic Act was passed by the United States Congress and the Act called for definitions of cosmetics and drugs.

2. ____ The FDA does not "approve" cosmetics.

3. ____ Cosmetic companies are required to list their products or formulas with the FDA.

4. ____ When a "bad" cosmetic is found by the FDA, they will have the company remove the cosmetic from the market immediately.

5. ____ The Food and Drug Act of 1938 defines drugs as "articles (other than food) intended to affect the structure or any function of the body that are intended to be rubbed, poured, sprinkled, or otherwise applied to the human body or any part thereof for cleansing, beautifying, promoting attractiveness or altering the appearance."

6. ____ The esthetician can state that a product will "shrink pores."

7. ____ The CTFA, or Cosmetics, Toiletries, and Fragrance Association, is the largest association of cosmetic manufacturers.

8. ____ The exception to the concentration rule of listing ingredients on a label according to concentration is when there is less than 1 percent of an ingredient.

9. ____ The sources of the ingredients are illegal to use on the ingredient label.

10. ____ Provided that it is true, claims that a product is FDA approved are legal.

11. ____ Active ingredients on an OTC (over-the-counter) product must list the active ingredients first with their purpose, and all other ingredients must be listed in the inactive ingredients section of the drug facts label.

Short Answer

1. A cosmetic that is claimed to be _____ has generally been manufactured without the use of ingredients that are known to frequently cause allergic reactions.
2. If a product is considered to be hypoallergenic, it does not necessarily mean that it is _____ because a person can be allergic to the ingredients contained within the product.
3. Treatment products that do not contain water are _____.
4. Preservative-free cosmetics have been recently developed as a result of _____ technology.
5. The term _____ means that ingredients that are known to cause comedone development and acne flare-ups have not been used in the cosmetic formula. The FDA does not require that _____ be performed to make a claim of _____.
6. When a product states that it has been "Dermatologist Tested" it does not necessarily mean that a product has been tested for all _____.
7. _____ cosmetics are not always superior to _____.
8. _____ literally means that the chemistry of a substance involves the element _____.
9. The term used to describe the way companies make their products sound better than they actually are is called _____.
10. Most ingredients have been tested on animals; however, in the future __ _____ testing may eliminate the need in favor of testing that occurs outside of a living _____.
11. The more _____ you have, the better you will be at _____ the most _____ companies from which to purchase products.
12. When purchasing products, the esthetician should do his or her _____ before buying from a company.
13. It's important to determine whether a company formulates products with _____ and _____ in mind and if they make claims about hypoallergenic or noncomedogenic products, whether they ____ their products.
14. It is also important to ask about the _____ history of a product line, who is the _____, and what are the credentials of the founder.

Define

Use the space provided to define these terms.

1. FDA

_____

_____

2. CTFA

_____

_____

3. Cosmeceutical

_____

_____

4. Anhydrous

_____

_____

5. Nonacnegenic

_____

_____

6. In vitro

_____

_____

Word Scramble

Unscramble the key terms below and write the term inside the cells, by using the definitions shown.

taclmceoseicu

- - - - - - - - - - - - - - - - - -   is a product designed for improving appearance but may have positive physiological effects on the skin, on a cellular level.

nepoalchlerygi

- - - - - - - - - - - - - - - - - -   cosmetics have generally been manufactured without the use of certain ingredients that are known to frequently cause allergic reactions.

dasnrhoyu

- - - - - - - - - - - - - - - - - -   treatment products that do not contain water.

vt irion

- - - - - - - - - - - - - - - - - -   refers to scientific testing that occurs outside of a living organism. It has not been tested on a live specimen.

liamc taannssubttiio gintste

- - - - - - - - - - - - - - - - - -   is performed, usually by independent consumer testing laboratories, to back up and document claims made by product companies.

Word Puzzle

It is important to be able to recognize different terms that describe claims, and the organizations that handle regulations involving cosmetics. See if you can find terms related to claims in cosmetics in the following word search. (*Hint:* the terms are also used in the word scramble above.)

```
G F C Q A Y W Y A C P A P U A D F T E
R G T O T D P H H L R G T O T D P H L
B Z T F R Y K H R A N H Y D R O U S M
F T E Q S A G A H I A D T A R P M G G
H H L M D S C O S M E C E U T I C A L
I B W B M L W P I S F O G H Y N G H R
L F P I U T A M M U F E G O E G Y R P
J I K W S X F H W B Y K L L A A L I K
G L Z R G U E W L S H S X F H H E M A
O H G R O G H Y G T L Z R G U E W L M
V H D V F G Y D M A R G F D F M H M H
A P I U T A M M F N C I K W S X F H W
H G R O G H Y N N T G M U T A T M A T
O E G Y R P S W D I Q K A Q A R Y A G
G H L D N C M E P A I G W A A L I K L
A K Y C Q K A Q Y T T Y K L W A A L W
Y K L L A A L I K I H G L Z R G U E W
L K R Q A F G K G O Z D V H D V F G Y
V G F G Q H L M D N Y L T A R P M G K
C G R H K C D F B T A G F L N H B Q D
P Z F E G O E G Y E R Q A R Y A M L F
K L W A A L I K L S L M W J E P I G O
A E L A D T I V T T T Y K L W A A O E
A L N B E L K R Q I N V I T R O M L F
G F D F M H M H A N R O E G Y R P S A
H Y P O A L L E R G E N I C O F I B W
```

CHAPTER 13

Sensitive Skin, Allergies, and Irritants

Multiple Choice

Circle the correct answer.

1. Sensitive skin is characterized as
   A. very thick, pink-colored skin with pigmented lesions.
   B. thin, fragile-looking, pink-colored skin on people with red or blond hair.
   C. thin, darker skin with telangiectasias present.
   D. skin that has many telangiectasias, often found on women with light skin and dark hair.

2. In sensitive skin, the blood vessels and nerve endings are closer to the surface as a result of the skin's
   A. sebaceous activity.   B. color.   C. thinness.   D. sensitivity.

3. Sensitive skin is becoming
   A. less prevalent.   B. easier to treat.   C. more common.   D. more difficult to treat.

4. Sensitive skin is most often
   A. Fitzpatrick I skin type.
   B. Fitzpatrick II skin type.
   C. Fitzpatrick III skin type.
   D. the type that burns but tans later.

5. Blanching is caused by
   A. tanning.   B. redness.   C. pressing on thin skin.   D. using lighteners.

6. Clients with sensitive skin will report frequent bouts of redness, hives, and swelling, which are descriptions of the following terms, respectively:
   A. erythema, urticaria, and edema
   B. edema, blanching, itching
   C. itching, swelling, and redness
   D. erythema, blanching, and welts

7. An objective symptom is
   A. one that can be felt.
   B. one that can be easily treated.
   C. one that is not visible.
   D. one that is visible physically and possibly can be measured.

8. Subjective symptoms are
   A. felt, such as itching, stinging, or burning.
   B. never physically visible.
   C. those that can always be seen.
   D. felt and are measurable.

9. Scientists believe that chronic subjective symptoms are
   A. psychological.   B. physiological.   C. neurological.   D. subclinical.

10. A client who has experienced many sensitivities
    A. is anxious to try new products and treatments.
    B. will usually know what causes their sensitivities.
    C. is likely leery of trying new things and does not want to experience the problem again.
    D. will expect that you will solve his or her problems.

11. With a sensitive skin type, it is important to
    A. protect the barrier function of the skin.
    B. exfoliate.
    C. use impermeable ingredients.
    D. use propylene glycol as an ingredient in the client's skin health products.

12. State-of-the-art sensitive skin products are now being produced with
    A. chemical emulsifiers.
    B. desincrustation ingredients.
    C. physical emulsifiers.
    D. mechanical exfoliants.

13. The inflammation cascade is
    A. a series of chemical reactions within the skin that occur when the skin is in balance.
    B. a series of reactions within the skin that create telangiectasias.
    C. a series of chemical reactions that occur when the skin is irritated.
    D. when the skin is dermatographic.

14. Not all clients with telangiectasias
    A. are dermatographic.
    B. have high blood pressure.
    C. are Fitzpatrick I skin types.
    D. are sensitive.

15. One of the most important aspects of using an analysis technique
    A. is to be certain to make careful note of your observations, along with any pertinent information obtained from the client history form.
    B. is to recommend the best products for sensitive skin types.
    C. is to make a diagnosis for your client so that you may recommend appropriate treatment.
    D. is to determine whether the sensitive skin type has immune responses and reactions as a result of the lack of blood close to the skin's surface.

True/False

Write T for true and F for false in the space provided.

1. ____ Dermatitis is a term used by dermatologists to describe general skin inflammation.

2. ____ Contact dermatitis is another term for dermatitis.

3. ____ Allergic contact dermatitis is an inflammation from an allergy to a particular chemical or substance.

4. ____ An allergy is the body's rejection of a particular agent or substance, which the immune system has identified as a foreign invader.

5. ____ The term "overprocessed skin" usually means that the skin has been overexfoliated and the use of too many products containing exfoliants has created irritant reactions that are characterized by red, flaky, and uncomfortable skin.

6. ____ Ingredients such as SD alcohols, clay masks, and sulfur should not pose a problem for irritated skin.

7. ____ Mechanical exfoliants are excellent for sensitive skin.

8. ____ Essential oils and steaming are good for sensitive, irritated skin.

9. ____ Clients with overprocessed skin may have a concern about aging and quite possibly are using too many products at once.

10. ____ When a person develops a routine allergic response to a substance, the person has become sensitized to that substance.

11. ____ Histamines are drugs that combat rashes, itching, and hives.

12. ____ Hypoallergenic and nonallergenic are basically the same term.

13. ____ Fragrances are the number one cause of cosmetic allergies.

14. ____ Many essential oils have undergone very little scientific testing and may present major problems for those with sensitive skin.

15. ____ Natural botanical ingredients are less irritating on sensitive skin than many other types of product ingredients.

Fill in the Blank

Using the word bank below, fill in the blank to complete the sentence. The same word or phrase may be used more than once.

Word Bank

color agents	sensitive	formaldehyde	zinc oxide	salicylates
preservatives	UVA	phenoxyethanol	titanium dioxide	aspirin
formalin donors	allergies	parabens	physical sunscreen	30
lipstick	methylparaben	PABA (para-amino	absorbing	irritations
eye shadow	propylparaben	benzoic acid)	micronize	SD alcohol
D & C yellow	butylparaben	UVB	octinoxate	cream
D & C red	ethylparaben	padimate-O	octyl salicylate	water resistant
patch test	allergy-prone	padimate-A	broad-spectrum	

1. ____ ____ are used in skin-care products strictly for market appeal and generally have nothing to do with the function of the product.

2. Many clients with sensitive skin may have color agent allergies that are associated with _____ and ___ _____ makeup products. The most offending color agents seem to be _____ _____ and _____ ___.

3. The function of _____ is to keep harmful bacteria from contaminating products. Unfortunately, they can produce _____.

4. _____ _____ _____ and _____ are used in thousands of cosmetic formulations; it is estimated that 1 percent of the United States population is allergic to these _____.

5. Many preservatives work by emitting minute quantities of _____ known as _____ _____.

6. If you are treating a client with a known preservative allergy, it is best to perform a ____ ___ for all products to be used and have a variety of products with different preservative systems on hand.

7. Most people tolerate preservative ingredients, but for those with _____ or _____ skin they may be problematic.

8. _____ is a nonformaldehyde-releasing preservative and is often used with _____.

9. _____ is rarely used as a sunscreen ingredient because of its potential to cause skin allergy. _____ and _____ are chemical cousins of _____.

10. The two sunscreen ingredients that are least likely to cause allergies are _____ and _____ _____. These ingredients are _____ _____ agents because they work by reflecting the UVA and UVB rays rather than by _____ them. New technology has been developed to _____ these white, opaque ingredients; thus they look less powdery on the skin.

11. To make a more user-friendly product that is not thick, companies often will mix ___ ____ or _____ ____ with a different sunscreen such as _____ or ____ _____, which produces a lighter-weight product that always provides excellent _____ protection against the ____ and ____ sunrays.

12. Some people are allergic to _____, a group of chemicals related to salicylic acid. If your client tells you that she or he has an _____ allergy, they are not a candidate for using products with _____.

13. Sunscreens should be applied ___ minutes before going out in the sun.

14. Sunscreen _____ are often the result of applying the product on hot skin and by using gels containing _____. It is best to use a _____ -based sunscreen because these have proven to be more ____ _____.

Matching

Match the term with the best description, and write the letter of the term in the space provided.

Description

1. ____ Red, flaky, swollen upper and lower eyelids.

2. ____ Clients who are allergic to jewelry, fabric softeners, and hard water may experience this.

3. ____ Products in which padimate-O, oxybenzone, and methyl salicylate may be found.

4. ____ Ingredients such as methylparaben, propylparaben, imidazolidinyl urea, quaternium-15, and triclosan.

5. ____ Salicylic acid and alpha hydroxy acids such as glycolic, lactic, malic, and tartaric acid are examples.

6. ____ Used for lightening the skin as in hyperpigmented lesions.

7. ____ Examples such as clove oil, cinnamics, eucalyptus, and geraniol.

8. ____ An ingredient used to make eye shadow appear frosted that can irritate sensitive eyelids.

9. ____ An alternative to benzoyl peroxide for acne, which can be a source of irritation to clients who are prone to allergies.

10. ____ A difficult combination of conditions to treat with sensitive skin.

11. ____ Allergens that are well known for possible allergic reactions or irritations.

12. ____ The best way to use effective, yet potentially irritating, ingredients on sensitive skin by alternating with a soothing product and decreasing the strength.

13. ____ Is excellent for acne in the 2.5 percent strength for sensitive skin.

14. ____ Clients can confuse this with irritants.

15. ____ Eyelid allergies and irritations can be created by this product.

16. ____ Alpha hydroxy acid products should have a pH no lower than this for sensitive skin types.

Terms

A. nail products

B. allergies

C. 3.5

D. acne and sensitive skin

E. minimize exposure

F. benzoyl peroxide

G. sulfur

H. mica

I. common allergens

J. fragrances

K. preservatives

L. sunscreens

M. exfoliants

N. noncosmetic allergies

O. eyelid dermatitis

P. hydroquinone

Short Answer

1. One of the most important basic concepts in treating sensitive skin is to be careful about protecting the _____ _____ of the skin.

2. Avoiding known _____ and _____ materials, products, and procedures that may cause an allergic or irritant reaction is also essential in treating a client with sensitive skin.

3. Use products and treatments that have low _____ _____.

4. Ingredients such as _____ _____, cornflower extract, _____ _____, _____, stearyl glycyrrhetinate, dipotassium glycyrrhetinate, *Matricaria* extract, and azulene have been shown to decrease sensitivity.

5. _____ _____ _____ is known as a 48-hour patch test, which involves applying a small amount of the product on the back of the test participant and then covering it with a bandage to be checked for irritation 2 days later.

6. A _____ ____ ____ _____ is considered more reliable by physicians and scientists to determine allergy or sensitivity potential of a given substance. This test is repeated at intervals, giving the immune system time to develop antibodies to the material being tested, which will likely reveal delayed allergy responses.

7. It is advisable when treating clients with sensitive or redness-prone skin to avoid ____, _____, and aggressive _____ _____.

8. Sensitive skin is best treated with _____ _____ ___ ____, a light, gentle, bead-type exfoliant, and gentle _____ using the _____ ____ technique. Once the skin has cooled, apply a ____ _____ massage, then apply a nonfragranced hydrating fluid and a _____ designed for _____ skin.

9. If a client experiences an extreme or severe reaction to a treatment or product, always refer them to a _____ immediately.

10. Clients with sensitive skin are to avoid ____ ___ _____, scrubs, and strong _____. Some clients with sensitive skin who also have rosacea may experience more redness while drinking _____ _____ and eating ____ ____.

Define and Briefly Discuss the Following

1. Sensitive skin cleansers

_____

_____

_____

_____

_____

2. Sensitive skin toners

_____

_____

_____

_____

_____

3. Antioxidants

_____

_____

_____

_____

_____

4. Sunscreens

_____

_____

_____

_____

5. Hydrators and moisturizers

_____

_____

_____

_____

6. Consultations with a client with sensitive skin

_____

_____

_____

_____

_____

_____

_____

_____

_____

7. External factors that influence sensitive skin

_____

_____

_____

_____

_____

_____

_____

_____

_____

_____

Word Scramble

Unscramble the key terms below and write the term inside the cells, by using the definitions shown.

hginanbcl

- - - - - - - - - - - - - - - -   occurs when the skin turns white upon being touched firmly with the fingers.

maeerthy

- - - - - - - - - - - - - - - -   refers to any area of redness associated with a lesion.

aartcriiu

- - - - - - - - - - - - - - - -   or hives, is due to allergies.

rrupsitu

- - - - - - - - - - - - - - - -   is the technical term for itching.

mlbeeapre

- - - - - - - - - - - - - - - -   means "easily penetrated."

harteeirdy

- - - - - - - - - - - - - - - -   describes a trait or condition inherited from parents; genetic.

artenstin

- - - - - - - - - - - - - - - -   means "temporary."

cyleesktuo

- - - - - - - - - - - - - - - -   are white blood cells.

nctykoei

- - - - - - - - - - - - - - - -   is a chemical released by cells to signal other chemical immune responses.

tspsoerae

- - - - - - - - - - - - - - - -   are enzymes that dissolve proteins.

bcinsuallci

- - - - - - - - - - - - - - - -   symptoms, such as stinging or tingling, have no visible appearance.

gredrpmtoaahci

- - - - - - - - - - - - - - - -   literally means "skin writing." Skin turns red and swells at the slightest scrape.

rdmeattsii

- - - - - - - - - - - - - - - -   means "inflammation of the skin."

gearlyl

- - - - - - - - - - - - - - - -   is the immune system's rejection of a particular substance.

ratintri

- - - - - - - - - - - - - - - -   is a substance that can inflame the skin.

tamnhsiei

- - - - - - - - - - - - - - - -   is a hormone-like chemical released during allergic reactions.

anmiessthiian

------------------   are drugs produced to combat the formation of histamines.

bbaoisoll

------------------   is an agent that is added to cosmetics designed for sensitive skin.

aleeunz

------------------   is a hydrocarbon derived from the chamomile flower.

nanciceeg

------------------   refers to the tendency of a product or ingredient to irritate the follicle, which can cause sudden flares of pimples.

ingccomdoee

------------------   is the tendency of a topical substance to cause a buildup of dead cells, resulting in the development of comedones.

ocotpalilergh

------------------   describes drugs that can cause allergic reactions if the patient has sun exposure while using the drug.

Word Puzzle

It is important to recognize and understand the terminology related to skin allergies and reactions. See how many related terms you can find in the following word search. (*Hint*: the terms are also used in the word scramble above.)

```
X F H H E M A L A D E W Q P H O T O A L L E R G I C Q G A U T A M M
K L T A O L I A D F O T H R Z H T G S H V Q H L M Y K A Q A R Y A G
L A A L I K L K C L I K K U D Y D S U T R B G K Y T O G H Y N O S D
I K W S X F H G Y A X A G R T H F Y D R U E M L W O H L D N C M E P
Q G A U T G A C N E G E N I C G L L F N S Z M S B K O E G Y R P S W
W D T D P H L O M D T D T T O M A J G C A N T I H I S T A M I N E S
A F K F F Y K M H R C F K U B M K M R R Y L T A R N M F G Q H L M D
Q L A G Q H L E M D S G A S F G H Q U T L K R Q A E R C R B G K Y C
H A D R B G K D Y C O R D T W L A R S M F L N H B Q G W U E M L W Y
K K C U E M L O W Y G U C U D E Q A C U H K C D F B F R Y K H R C G
G Y U S Z R S G B C M S Y C E K M A Z U L E N E Q G Z Q H L M D S F
X A T V D A H E R E D I T A R Y A L I K E A F P K A R B G K Y C O G
Z G W A G T X N F B P K A Q M K W S X F U Y E W O G U E M L W Y G R
A L A Q U R T I C A R I A H A G A U T G K H E M A R Y A M S B C M U
M F Q H A F Q C T F R Y K H T C Q A R A O G F L N H B Q D Q G A U S
K K H D G K H G F G Q H L M O S H Y B G C R H K C D F B P K A Q A B
A W K G L W K R C R B G K Y G O G A L T Y G L L R G U E W O G H Y F
W M G A E M G H E U E M L I R R I T A N T T K F S X F H H E M A N U
M D A L A L L E R G Y M S B A M D P N L E D A G Y K L M A Z L I U F
D R G U O T Q W Y D G K H G P A F R C K S R D R L D A Z L I K L A L
T R A N S I E N T G L W K R H W D Q H L M D C U J I K W S X F H Y A
M F Q H A F Q R H I S T A M I N E B I K Y C U S M Q G A U T G A N K
P E R M E A B L E P H L M D C R R E N L W Y T V Q K A Q A R A Q Y G
D G Y G R M I L M F Y K H R C W M Z G S B C W A R O G H Y N G H U A
F H U B A R S K A Q H L M D S E A A C U H K A Q V M Q G A U T A M G
L P P M F W A L R B G K Y P R O T E A S E S Q H A Q K A Q A R Y A Q
A E O J U E B K M E M L W Y G D I W A A L I K L G R O G H Y N O S K
K R E R T T O Y C Z M S B C M A T I K W S X F H A G H L D N C M E O
G V S U B C L I N I C A L M T I I Q G A U T G A E G O E G Y R P S H
A W R R P J O L R A G M R V A R S K A Q A R A Q M L F P I U T A M O
G B Q G R Z L B J F K Q M I W J T O G H Y N G H O F I B W B M L W F
```

CHAPTER 14

Rosacea

Multiple Choice

Circle the correct answer.

1. Rosacea is a common disorder of the skin associated with
   A. blackheads, cystic acne, and pigmentation.
   B. hyperpigmentation, spider veins, and sebaceous cysts.
   C. diffuse redness, acne-like papules, pustules, and dilated capillaries.
   D. diffuse redness, hyperpigmentation, and blackheads.

2. Rosacea was formerly known as
   A. acne vulgaris.
   B. adult acne.
   C. a disorder caused by the sun.
   D. couperose.

3. Clients with rosacea will often report symptoms of
   A. flushing and heat.
   B. hot and cool sensations.
   C. flushing and pigmentation changes.
   D. swelling and pigment changes.

4. Rosacea is a
   A. sinus disorder.
   B. disorder of the melanocytes.
   C. vascular disorder.
   D. vascular disease.

5. In clients with rosacea, the sudden rushing of blood to the facial skin can stimulate the
   A. sudoriferous glands.
   B. adrenal glands.
   C. lymph glands.
   D. sebaceous gland.

6. Vascular growth factor (VGF)
   A. triggers growth or expansion of new blood vessels, specifically the arterial capillaries.
   B. triggers activity in the lymph fluid.
   C. is something that we only see in adults older than age 50 years.
   D. triggers pigment and creates telangiectasias in the dermis of the skin.

7. The exact cause of rosacea is
   A. excessive drinking of alcohol.
   B. a person's diet.
   C. unknown at this time.
   D. a person's propensity to blush.

8. The topical medication often used to treat rosacea is
   A. antibiotic and isotretinoin.
   B. a natural extract of chamomile.
   C. a product containing essential oils.
   D. an antiyeast, antifungal.

9. When flares of rosacea are under control for long periods of time, this is referred to as
   A. remission.
   B. reoccurrence.
   C. reduction.
   D. cured.

10. *Demodex folliculorum* is known as
    A. a medication to manage rosacea.
    B. a type of yeast that has been theorized to cause rosacea.
    C. an intestinal bacterium found to cause rosacea.
    D. a mite, which has been theorized as a cause of rosacea.

True/False

Write T for true and F for false in the space provided.

1. ____ Rosacea is curable.

2. ____ Rosacea is often created by emotional turmoil.

3. ____ A rosacea flare can be caused by eating spicy foods or drinking a glass of red wine.

4. ____ Sun exposure can be responsible for rosacea flares in all people.

5. ____ Rosacea flares create an inflammation in the sebaceous glands.

6. ____ Stimulating skin-care products are recommended in the management of rosacea.

7. ____ It is necessary to avoid granular or rough scrubs for the skin health of clients with rosacea.

8. ____ Skin-care products containing fragrances should pose no problem for patients with rosacea.

9. ____ In general, the same precautions that are taken for rosacea should be taken for sensitive skin.

10. ____ Any form of heat or extreme cold can trigger flushing.

Fill in the Blank

Using the word bank below, fill in the blank to complete the sentence. The same word or phrase may be used more than once.

Word Bank

National Rosacea Society	papulopustular	phymatous	diagnosis	clogged pores
14 million	rhinophyma	four subtypes	estheticians	comedones
erythematotelang-iectatic	transient erythema	hordeolums	facial swelling	thickened
	ocular	granulomatous	dry patches	enlargement
	chalazia	dermatologist	grainy texture	

1. The _____ _____ _____ is a nonprofit organization founded for research, education, and support of people who have rosacea.

2. The Society estimates that as many as __ _____ Americans have some form of rosacea.

3. An expert committee of the Society has divided rosacea into ___ _____ of rosacea.

4. _____ rosacea is subtype 1 and is characterized by diffused facial redness, patchy redness on the nose and cheeks, and turning red easily.

5. A client who has redness that comes and goes may have _____ _____, which may also include ____ _____, __ _____, and ____ _____.

6. papulopustular rosacea is subtype 2, and it often resembles acne. The difference is there are no _____ ____ or _____ present.

7. Subtype 3 is called _____ rosacea. It has a _____ appearance and results in the _____ of the nose or other facial features.

8. _____ is the condition that creates an enlarged, bulbous nose that is often erroneously associated with alcoholism.

9. Subtype 4 occurs in the eyes and eyelids of patients, resulting in swollen lids. It is called _____ rosacea.

10. _____ are small, lumpy cysts in the eyelids, and _____ are better known as styes.

11. Although not a subtype, it causes hard, nodular papules in the cheeks and around the mouth; it is known as _____ rosacea.

12. As a medical condition, the _____ of rosacea must be left up to a physician, preferably a _____.

13. Physicians can rely on well-trained _____ for educating, providing esthetic and appearance support, and explaining proper skin care for their patients with rosacea.

Short Answer

1. _____ is a term for increased blood flow from dilated blood vessels, resulting in flushing or a rosacea flare.

2. There are many ways to _____ and _____ rosacea.

3. It is possible to keep the symptoms under control for long periods of time through the use of _____ _____ and _____ and _____ changes.

4. Rosacea flares and triggers are associated with ___ _____ _____, and _____.

5. The most common topical treatment drug for rosacea is _____, commercially known as Metrogel®, Metrolotion®, Metrocream®, or _____ . Under the names of Klaron® are _____ and _____ _____. One of the newest topical drugs for rosacea is called _____ , with 15 percent azelaic acid.

6. All of the prescription topical drugs for rosacea have _____ effects.

7. In addition to topical drugs, oral antibiotics such as _____ _____, and _____ may be prescribed for patients experiencing "flares" with their rosacea. In extreme cases of rosacea, _____ may be prescribed.

8. The goal in medical treatment of rosacea is to _____ inflammation and flares and, in some cases, ___ bacteria associated with papules and _____ .

9. Patients with rosacea may also suffer from _____ _____, a disorder caused by inflammation of the sebaceous gland, which may include _____ and _____ in oily areas such as the _____, hairline, and sides and corners of the ____.

10. Technological advancements have made it possible for patients with rosacea to have ____ and light therapies such as _____ and _____ for help with redness and the progression of rosacea at all levels.

Describe, Detail, or Name the Following

1. Detail the seven specific symptoms of rosacea

   A. _____

   B. _____

   C. _____

   _____

   D. _____

   _____

   E. _____

   F. _____

   G. _____

   _____

2. Describe the recommended skin products for clients with rosacea.
   A. Cleansers

   _____

   _____

   _____

   _____

   B. Toners

   _____

   _____

   _____

   _____

   C. Moisturizers

   _____

   _____

   _____

   _____

   D. Sunscreens

   _____

   _____

   _____

   _____

   E. Exfoliants

   _____

   _____

   _____

   _____

   F. Soothing products

   _____

   _____

   _____

   _____

   G. Medication

   _____

   _____

   _____

   _____

3. Describe a step-by-step home-care recommendation for a client with rosacea.

Morning

A. _____

B. _____

C. _____

D. _____

E. _____

F. _____

Evening

A. _____

B. _____

C. _____

D. _____

E. _____

4. Name eight treatment contraindications for clients with rosacea.

A. _____

B. _____

C. _____

D. _____

E. _____

F. _____

G. _____

H. _____

Word Scramble

Unscramble the key terms below and write the term inside the cells, by using the definitions shown.

insfluhg

------------------ refers to the reddening of the skin due to stimulation.

tleingesesaact

------------------ are dilated or distended capillaries.

anasiatelectgi

------------------ is a single distended capillary.

proscouee

------------------ refers to small, red, enlarged capillaries of the face and other areas of the body.

aslcravu

------------------ means "blood vessel related."

ondiltivaoas

------------------ is the dilation of the blood vessels, resulting in flushing.

issiomnre

------------------ is a phase of disease where the disease is dormant and no symptoms are present.

inoapmryhh

------------------ is an enlarging of the nose, often resulting from a severe form of acne rosacea.

zhlcaaai

------------------ are small, lumpy cysts in the eyelids.

deolhormus

------------------ or styes, are infected tear ducts.

oniodatrlemez

------------------ is a medication used to control rosacea and decrease inflammation.

lusrfu

------------------ is a topical drug agent used to treat rosacea.

teatlrcneicy

------------------ is an oral antibiotic used to treat more severe rosacea and other acne-related conditions.

yxloccneidy

------------------ is an oral antibiotic used to treat more severe rosacea.

cliynoiemnc

------------------ is an oral antibiotic used to treat more severe rosacea and other acne-related conditions.

omphoodulatinto

------------------ is the process of using light to treat conditions of the skin.

Word Puzzle

Understanding the terms associated with the common skin condition rosacea is important to estheticians. See how many terms related to rosacea you can find in the following word search. (*Hint*: the terms are also used in the word scramble above.)

```
X F H H E M A L P H F H F P K A R B G K Y C O
K L T A O L M I N O C Y C L I N E E M L W Y G
L A A L I K L K A R O G E M A R M A M S B C M
I K W S P H O T O M O D U L A T I O N Q G A U
Q G A H T G A C H A Q K H K C D S B P A M Q A
W D T U P H L H O R D E O L U M S E W T G H Y
A F K A H Y K M A W S X K F S X I G H R M A N
M L S Y Q H R E G A C O U P E R O S E N L I U
E A U R B G H D M Q H R D R L D N Z L U K L A
T E L A N G I E C T A S I A J I K W S X F H Y
R Y F S Z R N G K U L K U S M Q G A U T G A N
O A U V D A O E F D A O T V Q K A Q A R A Q Y
N G R A G T P N G F Z E W A R O G H Y N G D U
I L A Q U R H I A G I Z A Q V V Q G A U T O M
D F Q H A F Y C G V A S C U L A R A Q A R X A
A K H D G K M G T U T G K L G S O G H Y N Y S
Z W K G L W A R R D P H F H G O H L D N C C E
O M G A E M G H N F H Y G A E D O E G Y R Y S
L H I S T A T E T R A C Y C L I N E I U T C M
E E P H L M D C R R E W S X F L R B G K Y L G
L M F Y K H R C W M Z A U T G A M E M L W I A
K A Q H L M D S E A A Q A R A T C Z M S B N G
L R B G K Y P R O T E L A N G I E C T A S E S
K M E M L W Y G D I W A R Y A O G H Q U T L K
Y C Z M S B C M A F L U S H I N G A R S M F L
```

CHAPTER 15

Acne and the Esthetician

Multiple Choice

Circle the correct answer.

1. The most common form of acne is
   A. level 1.
   B. retention hyperkeratosis.
   C. acne vulgaris.
   D. noninflammatory acne lesion.

2. Acne is a condition that results in
   A. multiple breakouts.
   B. inflammatory and noninflammatory lesions.
   C. inflammatory lesions.
   D. hyperkeratosis.

3. A microcomedo is
   A. a noninflammatory lesion that is not red or inflamed.
   B. visible to the naked eye.
   C. a pustule.
   D. a small impaction formed by cells that have built up on the inside of the follicle wall.

4. Ostium refers to
   A. the hair follicle.
   B. the matrix of the hair.
   C. the bottom of the hair follicle.
   D. the opening in the follicle.

5. *Propionibacterium acnes* (*P. acnes*) is the scientific name of bacteria that cause
   A. acne vulgaris.
   B. comedones.
   C. hyperkeratosis.
   D. noninflammatory lesions.

6. The two major hereditary factors in acne development are
   A. retention hyperkeratosis and oiliness.
   B. melanin and retention hyperkeratosis.
   C. oiliness and melanin.
   D. "cell buildup" and open comedones.

7. A red, sore, surface bump without a "whitehead" is known as a
   A. cyst.
   B. pustule.
   C. papule.
   D. nodule.

8. A clump of white blood cells that have formed and risen to the surface of the skin is called a
   A. pustule.
   B. *Propionibacterium acnes*.
   C. microcomedo.
   D. noninflammatory lesion.

9. Grade 1 acne is
   A. commonly referred to as cystic acne, with many deep cysts and scar formation.
   B. mostly open and closed comedones with an occasional pimple.
   C. thought of as "typical teenage acne."
   D. skin with a very large number of closed comedones with occasional papules or pustules.

10. The hormone(s) often responsible for oily skin and acne is (are)
    A. estrogen.
    B. progesterone.
    C. the male hormones: androgens, testosterone, and dihydrotestosterone (DHT).
    D. a combination of estrogen and progesterone.

11. Both female and male hormones are transported in the body by
    A. fat.
    B. lymph fluid.
    C. estrogen.
    D. blood.

12. Perifollicular inflammation is
    A. an inflammation around the inside of the follicle.
    B. noninflammatory acne.
    C. a microcomedo.
    D. an increase in oxygen in the follicle.

13. Stress can bring about acne flare-ups because of the additional hormones made by the
    A. sebaceous glands.   B. adrenal glands.   C. sudoriferous glands.   D. lymph glands.

14. Many women notice that premenstrual flares can result in
    A. more comedones.   B. more microcomedones.   C. more inflammatory lesions.   D. more noninflammatory lesions.

15. A condition in which the skin exhibits redness and irritation in patches, accompanied by a rough texture and small pinpoint white bumps that look like tiny milia, is known as
    A. retention hyperkeratosis.   B. hyperkeratosis.   C. keratosis.   D. keratosis pilaris.

True/False

Write T for true and F for false in the space provided.

1. ____ The elevation in testosterone in a woman who is premenstrual is not so much an increase, but rather a decrease in estrogen.

2. ____ When heat and humidity are high, acne is more likely to flare up.

3. ____ Sun damage is documented to cause more "cell buildup," which can increase the chances of acne flare-ups.

4. ____ As an esthetician, it is important to train clients to tan only for the time that it takes to clear up acne.

5. ____ If an acne-prone client works in an oily or greasy environment, he or she should be cleansing his or her face twice during an 8-hour shift.

6. ____ In extreme cases of acne excoriée, the esthetician should try to determine how best to help the client by using peels and microdermabrasion.

7. ____ Post-inflammatory hyperpigmentation is caused by trauma to the skin.

8. ____ Some milk and milk products have been found to cause acne because of the hormones present in the milk.

9. ____ Chocolate and pizza cause acne.

10. ____ Estheticians should counsel clients on diet and offer advice on what supplements and medications to take.

11. ____ Perioral dermatitis is not considered an acne-related disorder.

12. ____ Seborrheic dermatitis is a chronic inflammation of the skin associated with oily skin and oily areas and is characterized by dry-looking, flaky, crusty patches.

13. ____ Hydrocortisone and salicylic acid are often used to treat seborrheic dermatitis.

14. ____ A chemical peel should be administered when a client has a flare of seborrheic dermatitis.

15. ____ The best treatment for perioral dermatitis is oral antibiotics.

Fill in the Blank

Using the word bank below, fill in the blank to complete the sentence. The same word or phrase may be used more than once.

Word Bank

follicular exfoliants	keratolytics	red	solidified sebum	erythromycin
adapalene	azelaic acid	resorcinol	exfoliating	acne
masks	microcomedones	antimicrobials	glycolic acid	microcomedo
every day	barrier function	cell buildup	clindamycin	tretinoin
benzoyl peroxide	sulfur	sensitive	cure	home-care products
tazarotene	comedogenic products	salicylic acid	sebum	
aspirin enzymes	exfoliate	antibiotics	lactic acid	

1. Treatment products for acne may include _____ _____, which works well on most forms of acne vulgaris and occasional pimples by peeling the excess cell buildup, temporarily dilating the follicles, and thus breaking up the follicle impactions.

2. _____ and _____ are often combined in an acne-drying product, such as a ____, and are usually less irritating than _____ _____.

3. One of the mildest of the drying agents is _____ ___; however, some clients are allergic to it. If your client is allergic to _____, avoid using _____ ___.

4. The primary lesion of acne is the _____. The key to controlling _____ is the daily use of _____ _____.

5. The real value in using follicular exfoliants is to _____, break up ___ _____ and _____ _____, and dry visible acne lesions with everyday use to keep the material from accumulating.

6. Although there is no ____ for ____, prevention is highly recommended by using appropriate home-care products ____ ___, even if a client's skin is perfectly clear.

7. _____ are not scrub cleansers, and they work by causing dead skin cells to shed by loosening them from each other. The most common OTC drug forms of these exfoliants are _____ _____ _____ _____, and _____ ___.

8. Exfoliant performance ingredients include _____ _____ and other alpha and beta hydroxy acids, and _____.

9. Prescription keratolytics include _____ (Tazorac®), and _____ (Azelex®). For clients using these prescriptions, it is important to not use more than one type of _____ agent at a time to avoid stripping the _____ _____ and making the skin ___ and _____.

10. _____ contain fatty agents and must be avoided when treating any skin that is already overproducing _____.

11. Drug chemicals that kill bacteria are known as _____ and _____. Prescription topical antibiotics include _____ and _____.

12. Scrubs and washes are very popular _____ _____ for clients, as are toners and astringents, a lightweight sun-protection product, a night treatment including peeling agents, and _____. As always, caution should be taken not to over-treat the skin, making it _____.

Short Answer

1. _____ is an oil-absorbing clay frequently used in clay cleansing masks.

2. Home care for beginning teenage acne should include a _____ foaming cleanser.

3. Alpha hydroxy acid used daily for teenage acne should be between _ and __ percent to prevent the development of microcomedones.

4. A lightweight broad-spectrum sunscreen should be used daily with an SPF of no less than __ on teenage skin with acne because most sun damage occurs before the age of __.

5. Teenagers will often perform home care better if they do not feel _____.

6. Home care for treatment of Grade 1 acne should include cleansing _____ a day and applying alpha hydroxy acid _____ a day and _ percent benzoyl peroxide to all clogged and oily areas at night. A lightweight _____ with an SPF of 15 should always be used during the day.

7. Grade 2 acne is one of the _____ types to clear, and treatments in the salon should be _____ or _____.

8. Most Grade 3 acne cases should be seen by both the _____ and the _____. This client will often be placed on ___ _____ by a physician.

9. The care for a Grade 4 acne client always requires a visit to a _____. This is the _____ condition of acne and usually results in some type of _____.

10. Retin-A®, Differin®, and Tazorac® are all derivatives of vitamin A acid, and are prescription drugs that work by clearing the _____ of debris.

11. _____ is made from azelaic acid, which helps to _____ out follicular debris and has been found to act as a _____ suppressant.

12. All clients placed on retinoids and other prescription exfoliants should not use highly _____ cleansers, _____, and _____, and they should use a lightweight sunscreen with an ___ of 30 because these preparations will make their skin more photosensitive.

13. _____ is a form of retinoic acid and is prescribed for patients with severe acne. It has numerous ___ _____, and periodic _____ _____ is required to make certain that the body's organs are not being affected by the drug.

Describe, Define, or Detail the Following

1. Describe the precautions the esthetician should take with a client taking Accutane®.

_____

_____

_____

_____

_____

_____

_____

_____

_____

_____

_____

2. Describe a dermatological treatment for cysts.

_____

_____

_____

_____

3. Detail photodynamic therapy for acne.

_____

_____

_____

_____

_____

_____

4. Define seborrheic dermatitis.

_____

_____

_____

5. Define the use of glycolic and other chemical peels for acne.

_____

_____

_____

6. Define contraindications for treating a client with a chemical peel.

_____

_____

_____

_____

_____

_____

_____

Word Scramble

Unscramble the key terms below and write the term inside the cells, by using the definitions shown.

enca

-------------------- is a skin condition that results in inflammatory and noninflammatory lesions.

itaryheerd

-------------------- means a trait or condition is inherited from the parents; it is genetic.

lioessin

-------------------- describes a larger-than-normal amount of sebum secreted onto the skin by the sebaceous glands.

iromemccodo

-------------------- is a small impaction formed by cells that have built up on the inside of the follicle wall.

madelfni

-------------------- means "swollen and red."

rnoinnmlfaatomy

-------------------- refers to an impaction that is not red or inflamed.

iomstu

-------------------- is the opening in follicles.

icaanerob

-------------------- bacteria are those that do not need oxygen to grow and survive.

nmailne

-------------------- is the pigment of the skin.

eauplp

-------------------- is a raised area on the skin; it is generally smaller than 1 centimeter.

uspulte

-------------------- is a clump of white blood cells that have formed and risen to the surface of the skin.

eoldun

-------------------- is a raised lesion that is larger and deeper in the skin. A nodule looks like a lump, but the skin can be moved over the lesion.

etestoeronts

-------------------- is the male hormone responsible for the development of typical male characteristics.

flusru

-------------------- is an exfoliant and an antibacterial.

inorresclo

-------------------- is a peeling agent, usually coupled with sulfur, used in acne treatments and drying lotions.

zneesmy

-------------------- are naturally occurring chemical substances that help dissolve cell buildup.

taaroeenzt

------------------ is a topical prescription retinoid (vitamin A derivative) used to treat acne. It is commercially known as Tazorac®.

yertmhinrcoy

------------------ is an antibiotic used topically for medical acne treatment.

toibeennt

------------------ is an oil-absorbing clay frequently used in clay cleansing masks.

trinnoeit

------------------ is a form of vitamin A acid, also known as Retin-A®, a prescription drug for treating acne.

yclinindcma

------------------ is a topical prescription antibiotic used for acne treatment.

aapleenda

------------------ is a form of vitamin A, also known as Differin®, that is a topical prescription drug used for acne treatment.

Word Puzzle

It is important to understand terms related to acne and acne treatments. See if you can find acne and acne treatment-related terms in the following word search. (*Hint:* the terms are also used in the word scramble above.)

```
X P K A R B G K Y T R E T I N O I N B P K A Q G
E W O G U E M L W Y G D T D P H N B M D T D T Q
E M A R Y A M S B C M F K F F Y F F H R C F K K
F L N H B Q D Q G A U L N O D U L E M D S G A O
H K C D F B P K A Q G A D R B G A F Y C O R D T
L L R G U E W O G H Y K C U E M M L W Y G U C U
K F S X F H H E M A N Y U S Z R M A B C M S C C
A G Y K L M A Z L I U A T V D A A C N E A Z L I
D R L D A Z L I K L A G W A G T T G F B P K I Q
C U J I K W S X F H Y L T E S T O S T E R O N E
U S M Q G A U T P A N F A H A F R G T N R Y D H
T V Q K A Q A R A Q Y K Z D G K Y X F Z Q H A M
W A R O G H Y N P H U W A G L W K R C Y B G M Y
A Q V M Q G A S U L F U R R Y K H T C M A R Y B
Q H A Q K A Q A L Y A E O Q H L M O S E Y B C G
K L A D A P A L E N E Z T B O K Y G O S A L I A
F H G G H L D N C M E D E E I L I R R I T A N G
G A E G O R E S O R C I N O L S B A M D P N L M
A H M L F P R U T A M S E G I H G P A F O C K L
E E L W O H Y D N C Y G O G N L T Y G L S R G U
Z R S B K O T G Y R I R R B E N T O N I T E X F
N E I H I S H A M I B A M D S N L E D A I Y K L
L D A R N M R G M H G P P U S T U L E D U L D A
M I C R O C O M E D O H W D Q H L M D C M J I K
L T H B Q G M U L M M I N E B I K Y C U S M Q G
K A D F B F Y Y A N A E R O B I C W Y T V Q K A
E R E Q G Z C H N M R C W M Z G S B C W A R O G
A Y P K A R I G I Y D S E A A C U H K A Q V M Q
Y E W O G U N O N I N F L A M M A T O R Y A Q K
```

CHAPTER 16

Comedogenicity

Multiple Choice

Circle the correct answer.

1. Comedogenicity is
   A. multiple comedones, both open and closed, and inflammatory acne.
   B. the tendency of topical substances to cause the development of comedones, possibly leading to or worsening acne eruptions.
   C. a group of product ingredients that safeguard against clogging and plugging the pores.
   D. a topical substance that protects the skin from "cell buildup."

2. Acne that is caused or worsened by the use of comedogenic or inflammatory cosmetics or skin-care products is called
   A. noncomedogenic.
   B. perifollicular irritation.
   C. acnegenic.
   D. acne cosmetica.

3. Acnegenic reactions resulting from perifollicular irritation
   A. can take months to occur.
   B. can occur very quickly.
   C. are noninflammatory.
   D. are comedones.

4. Acne cosmetica looks like
   A. deeper cystic acne.
   B. sudden flares of inflammation.
   C. bumpiness just under the surface of the skin.
   D. hyperkeratosis.

5. Pomade acne is
   A. a type of acne associated with comedogenic pressing agents and dyes at the "blushline."
   B. flares of acne without comedones and can result from hormonal flares or acnegenic products causing follicle irritation.
   C. acne located in the T-zone.
   D. bumpiness in the skin of the forehead and around the hairline that is often caused by comedogenic or irritating hair products such as styling gels, conditioners, scalp oils, and sprays.

6. A histopathological study is
   A. a microscopic examination of tissue to determine causes of disease or abnormality.
   B. a study to determine how rapidly one develops retention hyperkeratosis.
   C. a biopsy.
   D. a microscopic study to determine the chemical makeup of a product or ingredient.

7. A synthetic polymer that is used in tissue sampling is called
   A. cyanoacrylate.
   B. a wax.
   C. fatty alcohol.
   D. an ester.

8. The best confirmation of noncomedogenicity and nonirritancy is
   A. to have the manufacturer conduct its own histopathological studies.
   B. to have all testing done on humans.
   C. to have documentation of testing by an independent test laboratory.
   D. for manufacturers to develop products using only the best product ingredients.

True/False

Write T for true and F for false in the space provided.

1. ____ Acne cosmetica is acne caused or worsened by the use of comedogenic or inflammatory cosmetics or skin-care products.

2. ____ Blushline acne is a type of acne cosmetica with multiple closed comedones in the blushline caused by comedogenic pressing agents and dyes in the blush.

3. ____ Scientists believe that human studies are more accurate and reliable in the evaluation of comedogenicity and follicle irritancy than rabbit ear studies.

4. ____ Spreading agents or vehicles are not comedogenic.

5. ____ All comedogenic ingredients feel heavy to the touch.

6. ____ It is important for estheticians to purchase products that have been tested by an independent laboratory to ensure that they are truly noncomedogenic and nonacnegenic.

7. ____ Petroleum is highly comedogenic.

8. ____ Fatty esters are often comedogenic.

Matching

Match the term with the best description, and write the letter of the term in the space provided.

Description   *Terms*

1. ____ Extracts, pigments, and humectants are noncomedogenic forms of these agents.   A. emollients

2. ____ Obtained from combining alcohols with fatty acids, these ingredients are often   B. oils
comedogenic.

3. ____ Used as emollients, these ingredients are less comedogenic than some acids.   C. fatty acids

4. ____ These ingredients are often derived from fats and waxes of animal or   D. fatty alcohols
vegetable origin and often are comedogenic.

5. ____ Peach kernel, linseed, grapeseed, and sesame are all highly comedogenic and   E. esters
are of this substance, be it vegetable or animal.

6. ____ These cosmetic chemicals give the product a creamy consistency and are   F. red dyes
highly comedogenic.

7. ____ Derived from sheep sebum, it becomes comedogenic when altered chemically.   G. performance
ingredients

8. ____ These ingredients are derivatives of coal tar, which is highly comedogenic.   H. lanolin

Short Answer

1. The _____ the molecule, the ___ likely the ingredient is to be comedogenic.

2. Some ____ ____ become less or more comedogenic when _____ _____.

3. When a large molecular structure is added to a fatty acid, it tends to become ___ comedogenic.

4. When fat is broken down, it becomes ____ _____.

5. In theory, the size of the _____ determines its ability to penetrate the follicle.

6. Known comedogenic ingredients should not be used in products that are designed for _____ ___ __ _____ skin.

7. _____ are added to talc and other products to create _____ or cake-type blush and powder.

8. _____ _____ _____ _____, and mineral oil are safe ingredients to use in pressed powders. They do not cause _____ and make good _____ _____.

9. Loose powders should be free of _____ _____ and ____ ___–derived D & C ___ ____.

10. Superfatted soaps are often made with ___ that can be _____ comedogenic.

11. Cleansers that are rinsable and do not leave a _____ on the skin are best for most skin types.

12. Sunscreens for oily skin are usually in a ____ _____ blended with _____ to guard against _____. They must be _____ screening for both _____ and _____ light rays. They must not be _____ or ___.

13. The two basic types of night treatments for clogged and problem skin are _____ and _____ products. Oily skin can still become _____, hence a _____ _____textured, _____ product must be used.

14. Ingredients such as _____ _____ _____ __ _____ will not clog acne-prone, problem skin.

15. Foundation for clogged and acne-prone skin should be _____ and in a _____ liquid.

16. Whereas _____ makeup is excellent because it is largely comprised of _____ ingredients, it may be compounded with a ____ substance to help it adhere to the skin. It should be checked for comedogenic _____ that are used as spreading agents, which may clog skin.

17. Hair conditioners and styling products often contain ____ ____ and other comedogenic _____ and must not be used on the skin.

18. Eye creams or concealers may ____ onto upper cheeks and may cause problems for acne-prone areas.

19. Many older women suffer from dehydrated skin that is also clogged, which is known as _____ skin. It may, in fact, be creating enough ___ underneath, yet is ___ on the surface. The tendency is to use products for _____ skin because these women are concerned with ____ . However, these products will create problems for _____ skin, when what the skin really needs is _____. That is _____ not ___.

20. Hydrating ingredients such as _____ ___ and _____ are good choices for the _____ client's skin. It is also important to avoid using _____ peeling _____ on these clients because their skin may feel more ___ to them. Make certain to _____ them as much as possible post-peel, and follow them closely while you ensure _____ with their new home-care program.

21. The two claims that are often made for products designed for oily skin are __ ___ and ____ ____. Neither of these terms mean _____. An oil-free product may contain _____ ___ ____, and other comedogenic ingredients.

Name, Detail, or Describe the Following

1. Name all products that should be checked during a comedogenic analysis.

_____

_____

_____

_____

_____

_____

_____

2. Detail an analysis procedure during a consultation with the client.

_____

_____

_____

_____

_____

_____

_____

_____

_____

_____

3. Describe which noncomedogenic ingredients you would want to see in the following products for a client who is acne prone and clog prone and why.

A. Cleanser: _____

_____

B. Toner: _____

C. Hydrator: _____

D. Sunscreen: _____

_____

Word Scramble

Unscramble the key terms below and write the term inside the cells, by using the definitions shown.

myegecoodnicit

- - - - - - - - - - - - - - - - - is the tendency of topical substances to cause the development of comedones, possibly leading to or worsening acne eruptions.

enca acometics

- - - - - - - - - - - - - - - - - is acne caused or worsened by the use of comedogenic or inflammatory cosmetics or skin-care products.

gecmooniced

- - - - - - - - - - - - - - - - - refers to the tendency of a topical ingredient or product to increase the buildup of dead cells within the follicle, eventually causing comedone formation.

cndooomegicenn

- - - - - - - - - - - - - - - - - means that the ingredient or product does not cause excessive follicular hyperkeratosis and therefore is unlikely to cause comedone development.

eganneicc

- - - - - - - - - - - - - - - - - refers to the tendency of a topical substance, usually a cosmetic or skin-care product, to cause inflammation or aggravate acne.

myinlaaorfmt eacn

- - - - - - - - - - - - - - - - - is flares of acne without comedones; it can result from hormonal flares or acnegenic products causing follicle irritation.

blueshinl enca

- - - - - - - - - - - - - - - - - is a type of acne cosmetica characterized by multiple closed comedones in the blushline; it is caused by comedogenic pressing agents and/or dyes in the blush.

ompaed eanc

- - - - - - - - - - - - - - - - - is bumpiness in the skin of the forehead and around the hairline.

tcghostiiphoalola

- - - - - - - - - - - - - - - - - refers to microscopic examination of tissue to determine causes of disease or abnormality.

edbiospi

- - - - - - - - - - - - - - - - - refers to removal of a small sample of tissue for microscopic or other examination.

yacaoclatenry

- - - - - - - - - - - - - - - - - is a synthetic polymer, commonly known as superglue.

lmneira pmaeku

- - - - - - - - - - - - - - - - - is another term for loose powder makeup foundation; it largely comprises earth-based ingredients. This product contains coverage pigments like zinc oxide and titanium dioxide, both of which are also physical sunscreens.

Word Puzzle

It is important to understand the terms associated with the causes of breakouts (comedones or acne flares, for example). See if you can find terms related to comedogenicity (comedone development) in the following word search. (*Hint:* the terms are also used in the word scramble above.)

```
K R H W D Q H L B M D C A J I H U I H D G K O G
A M I H N E B I L K Y C C U A S M N Q A MI N E
M D C I R R E N U L R R N I C T A F N T T K F S
X F M S D C R R S E N L E K N C D L F P K A N H
I K Y T C U S M H Q C N C R E Y C A M D C R R E
D S E O R O T Y L P Y R O O G T E M C W A R O P
M Y P P R O M S I O A M S U E M L M E I R R I N
W O G A H K C D N F N S M T N M S A U E E N E O
K E M T M C O M E D O G E N I C I T Y N E Q G N
M G K H H E M A A T A I T I C T I O F P K A Q C
K E A O I R R T C A C A I A R E B R K A R F U O
G A R L P C P R N W R O C K A R E Y F P K A R M
N A N O E O E A E A Y S A E P O MA D E A C N E
A K E G E M R O T P L R O T E S E C E A F P K D
F P M I N E R A L M A K E U P I R N Y P R O T O
C D F C E D H K E W T A N T T K F E K E A F P G
E E N A Q O Y E W O E I S E A A C U H E MA R E
N E Q L K G G K E I R R T A Y C U S M Q Y M E N
U L E N E E M Q K E A F P K A R F U Y E W O G I
T Y F P K N A K E A F P K A R E B I K Y C U S C
B I O P S I E D F U Y E W O G U G K H E MG A R
K F S X F C Y P R O T E A S E I R R I T N A N T
```

CHAPTER 17

Extraction

Multiple Choice

Circle the correct answer.

1. Extraction refers to
   A. removal of dead cells, sebum, bacteria, and other debris from the skin's follicles.
   B. an expulsion technique that is one of the most important functions of a facial.
   C. a treatment technique that, when omitted from a facial, may lead to acne, health problems, and possibly permanent scarring.
   D. all of the above.

2. A hereditary condition that refers to the tendency of dead skin cells to not shed in a regular and uniform manner and accumulate inside the follicle is called
   A. retention hyperkeratosis.
   B. open comedones.
   C. closed comedones.
   D. sebaceous filaments.

3. The first step in performing extractions is
   A. checking the perimeter of the face for acne lesions.
   B. cleansing the skin well.
   C. checking the skin for sebaceous filaments.
   D. scanning the "T-zone" for blackheads.

4. Sebaceous filaments indicate
   A. an open comedone.
   B. a closed comedone.
   C. an oily area.
   D. a dry area.

5. Before extracting it is important to
   A. presoften the accumulations in the skin.
   B. apply a glycolic peel.
   C. apply a cleanser to the skin.
   D. use a toner.

6. It is important to wear gloves
   A. during extractions.
   B. during the entire treatment.
   C. only if there are acne lesions present.
   D. at the beginning of the treatment.

7. The best extraction technique for extracting open comedones is using
   A. galvanic.
   B. high frequency.
   C. microdermabrasion.
   D. the cotton swab technique.

8. Closed comedones are most frequently found
   A. on the nose.
   B. on the forehead, neck, and chest.
   C. on the forehead.
   D. anywhere, but most often on the cheeks, jawline, and chin.

9. If you find a large number of closed comedones on the cheek area of a female client, it may be indicative of
   A. comedogenic reaction to blush.
   B. sebaceous filaments.
   C. retention hyperkeratosis.
   D. a moisturizing product being overused for aging skin.

10. Closed comedones are
    A. the easiest to extract.
    B. the most difficult to extract.
    C. dilated follicles.
    D. best extracted with the comedone extractor.

True/False

Write T for true and F for false in the space provided.

1. ____ In most closed comedones, follicle dilation is necessary.

2. ____ The cotton swab technique is best used on closed comedones.

3. ____ Favre-Racouchot is caused by sun exposure.

4. ____ Milia are rarely seen around the eye area.

5. ____ Milia will always have capillaries running through it.

6. ____ Xanthelasmas are flatter than milia and are yellow in appearance.

7. ____ Estheticians can easily remove xanthelasmas.

8. ____ Clients who do not remove their makeup at night are at risk for developing milia.

Short Answer

1. Extraction techniques require _____ training and really cannot be learned appropriately by studying a book.

2. Some states do not allow the use of _____ for extraction.

3. Almost every client's skin that you will see under the _____ ____ will need some _____.

4. _____ _____ are the small clogged pores many clients have on their ____.

5. It is important not to use a ____ after cleansing the skin because it will make the pores look _____ and will _____ them, preventing proper _____.

6. Holding the skin ___ between your _____ will make the skin easier to analyze and thus determine what needs to be extracted.

7. _____ is the process of _____ the skin and _____ _____ by applying a chemical that helps to _____ the sebum.

8. _____ solutions usually have a _____ or more _____ pH.

9. _____ ____ are used in a _____ manner to _____ comedones and _____ _____.

10. Some _____ are also used for loosening ____ ___ and _____ ____ on skin that is also dehydrated.

11. Using light peel treatments performed with _____ or _____ ___ can help to remove ____ _____ ___ _____.

12. Clients who have had at least ___ _____ __ ____ _____ ____ in their home-care program may have a __ _____ ____ _____ ___ peel at the beginning of their _____ treatment.

13. _____ the surface of the skin helps to _____ ____ ___ and helps to ____ _____ _____; however, it may not significantly affect the _____ _____ in the _____.

14. _____ products are designed to work on the ____ ____, whereas _____ and ____ _____ ____ work more on ____ ___ _____.

15. _____ should always wear _____ throughout the _____.

16. Extractions should not be _____ for more than __ _____ in one visit.

17. Clogged skin that has had more than 10 minutes of _____ should not be _____.

Detail and Define the Following

1. Detail some general rules for extraction.

   A. _____

   B. _____

   C. _____

   D. _____

   E. _____

   F. _____

   G. _____

2. Define examination procedures for extraction.

   A. _____

   B. _____

   _____

   C. _____

   _____

   D. _____

   _____

   E. _____

   F. _____

   G. _____

   _____

Word Scramble

Unscramble the key terms below and write the term inside the cells, by using the definitions shown.

---

treacnxito

- - - - - - - - - - - - - - - - - -   refers to the removal of dead cells, sebum, bacteria, and other debris from the skin's follicles.

treenoitn yperkaoerthssi

- - - - - - - - - - - - - - - - - -   refers to an overabundance of sebum that often begins at the time teenagers begin producing larger amounts of sex hormones.

becasouse ilmnasfet

- - - - - - - - - - - - - - - - - -   are small, impacted follicles on the nose and other facial areas; they are caused by oxidized, solidified sebum.

noep escmeoond

- - - - - - - - - - - - - - - - - -   are noninflammatory acne lesions, usually called blackheads.

ceosdl oconmedes

- - - - - - - - - - - - - - - - - -   are noninflammatory acne lesions, called whiteheads.

tomsiu

- - - - - - - - - - - - - - - - - -   is the opening in follicle.

piaidcli

- - - - - - - - - - - - - - - - - -   means "lack of lipids." These skin types do not produce enough lipids.

rudesttiscnanoi

- - - - - - - - - - - - - - - - - -   refers to the process of softening the skin and sebaceous impaction by applying a chemical that helps liquefy the sebum, reducing hard, solid plugs to a softer consistency.

liima

- - - - - - - - - - - - - - - - - -   are small deposits of sebum between the follicle and the corneum.

atxnelhmaass

- - - - - - - - - - - - - - - - - -   are much flatter than milia, have a yellowish appearance, are below the skin's surface, and may have an irregular shape.

grynomassi

- - - - - - - - - - - - - - - - - -   are small pinpoint lesions that occur under the eyes.

Word Puzzle

Recognizing and understanding the terminology related to extraction is just as important as finding the blemishes that need extracting. Find as many terms as you can related to extraction in the following word search. (*Hint*: the terms are also used in the word scramble above.)

```
D S U T C L Y S K K U D Y O D S U T M R B G K Y T O G B G O
F Y D R Y A E A G R T H F S Y D E S I N C R U S T A T I O N
L L F N N E B E N I C G L T L F N S L Z M S B K O E L L F N
A J G C M D A R D T T O M I A J G C I A N S I H I S T G K Y
K M R R H R S E B A C E O U S F I L A M E N T S A R S M Y C
C F K U B M K T M R R Y L M Y A R N M F A R S M Y C O S T I
H Q U T M D E E G A S F G H Q U T L K R Q A E R C A R S M Y
A R S M O P E N C O M E D O N E S Y C O S T I U M Q C C U W
Q C C U W Y U T U C U D E Q A C U H K N D F B A R M L Z U O
M Y C A L I P I D I C A R S M Y C A O I K P E I X A R Y A L
A R S M F D I O W A A R R E N L W Y T V E X T R A C T I O N
O S E A S N E N B I K Y C U S M Q G A I T G A N Y O S E A S
E S E A C S W H D Q H L M D C U J I K W L X F H Y M N L W Y
R Y O E N N M Y D P A L E D A G Y K L M M Z L I U E A R R E
E R T R W S X P F E B F K A Q M K W S X F U Y M W O G P E G
K I Y A R N M E X T R A C T I O N R C T A O R M G E Y G O G
C N A R S M Y R K F S X F H T K F E N L W Y T V X S X F H T
H G C U W Y U K K E I X A R Y A L Q C C U W Y U D S U T C L
A O Y C L O S E D C O M E D O N E S Y S A R R E N L W Y T V
Q M A R S M Y R O N T I E C F K U B M K C F K U B M K Z U O
X A N T H E L A S M A S A C M D E M N R C T A O R M G E Y G
M S Z U O C S T S Y C E K M A Z U L E G E Q G L Q C T A O R
M O P N M U E O M L I R R I T A N T T K F S X F H T K F S X
N D B I O R S S T M N T T K F S X F H H A T H A K F S X F H
N D B I O R S I T M N T T K F S X F H M E M N A T R O E N N
D I W A A R R S E N L W Y T V X F H N D B I O R S T M N T T
```

CHAPTER 18

The Intrinsic Aging Process

Multiple Choice

Circle the correct answer.

1. Extrinsic and intrinsic aging factors
   A. contribute to the outside influences of skin health.
   B. contribute to the inside influences of skin health.
   C. are preventable.
   D. contribute to the outside and the inside influences of aging, respectively.

2. Scientists believe that 85 percent of aging is the result of
   A. intrinsic aging factors.
   B. tanning.
   C. extrinsic aging factors.
   D. repetitive facial expressions.

3. Heredity plays a role in aging, and in general,
   A. the lighter the skin, the less visible aging will take place.
   B. the darker the skin, the less visible aging will take place.
   C. darker skin does not age.
   D. thicker skin shows age faster than thinner skin.

4. Elastosis means
   A. a loss of elasticity in the skin.
   B. an increase in elasticity in the skin.
   C. a loss of expression lines.
   D. skin that has lost fat.

5. Intrinsic aging can be fought by
   A. avoiding the sun.
   B. using the best skin-care products available.
   C. understanding how the skin functions.
   D. developing good health habits.

6. Although the esthetician does not give nutritional advice and counseling, he or she should
   A. have a working knowledge of the elements of nutrition to better direct the client to the proper, qualified professionals.
   B. have a working knowledge of proper nutrition to recommend supplementation such as antioxidants.
   C. have a working knowledge of proper nutrition to study health at the local community college or university.
   D. have a working knowledge of proper nutrition to recognize and treat those clients with a potential eating disorder.

7. Dehydration is known as
   A. skin that lacks nutrition.
   B. the decreasing ability of the skin to hold water.
   C. skin that is oil-dry.
   D. the increasing ability of the skin to hold water.

8. Wrinkles associated with intrinsic aging are primarily
   A. those caused by the sun.
   B. those caused by pollution and stress.
   C. expression lines.
   D. known as criss-cross wrinkling.

True/False

Write T for true and F for false in the space provided.

1. ____ Sagging associated with intrinsic aging is relatively minor and is attributable to gravity and intrinsic physiological changes.

2. ____ Criss-cross wrinkling not located in the regular facial expression along with severe elastosis is associated with intrinsic aging.

3. ____ There is nothing we can do about intrinsic aging.

4. ____ High levels of stress accelerate the aging process.

5. ____ Good skin-care habits are most effective when started any time in life.

6. ____ An increase in cell turnover occurs as the skin ages, resulting in uneven skin texture and a dull look to the skin.

7. ____ exfoliants, such as alpha hydroxy acids, remove dried-out, dull-looking, coarse skin, which will help the skin look smoother and more hydrated.

8. ____ Peptides have been shown to slow the signs of aging in the skin.

Fill in the Blank

Using the word bank, fill in the blank with the correct answer. Words may be used more than once.

Word Bank

extrinsic	mechanical exfoliants	overexfoliate	dilation	enzymes
antioxidants	"age spots"	elastin fibrils	palmitoyl	epidermis
internal	collagen	elasticity	pentapeptide-3	vasodilators
hyperpigmentation	solar damage	elastosis	esthetician	skin health
aging	heredity	alpha hydroxy acids	external	treatments
intrinsic	cell turnover			

1. Most people fear _____. The two major types of factors that contribute to _____ skin are _____ aging factors and _____ aging factors. _____ aging factors are those associated with _____ influences, and _____ aging factors are associated with _____ influences such as expression lines.

2. _____ is the cause of some aging factors, such as ethnicity and skin color. Darker skin tends to ward off more solar _____ than light skin.

3. Gravity plays a role on aging factors because even those with the best skin care and treatment will experience some _____, which means skin will have a loss of _____.

4. Good skin-care habits are most effective when started early to prevent problems by using daily sunscreens, _____, and ____ _____ ____ and having regular visits to an _____ for ___ _____ _____.

5. _____ _____ _____, and ____ _____ ____ help to increase ___ _____.

6. The _____ slowly becomes thinner with age. The breakdown of the network of _____ ___ _____ ____ within the dermis also occurs. _____ -stimulating peptides such as _____ _____ have been found to delaying the signs of aging.

7. Clients with older skin must be careful to not _____ by using harsh abrasives or applying too much pressure on their skin. In addition, they should avoid _____ such as alcoholic beverages, tobacco, and spicy foods because they cause _____ of the blood vessels and sudden surges of blood flow in the already fragile vessels.

8. Commonly called "_____," dark splotches or _____ are often one of the first signs of skin damage; they are caused by _____.

Define and Give Examples of the Following

1. Intrinsic aging factors

   _____

   _____

   _____

   _____

2. Extrinsic aging factors

   _____

   _____

   _____

   _____

3. Home-care exfoliation for aging skin

   _____

   _____

   _____

   _____

4. Skin treatments for aging skin

   _____

   _____

   _____

   _____

   _____

Word Scramble

Unscramble the key terms below and write the term inside the cells, by using the definitions shown.

---

tersinicx

- - - - - - - - - - - - - - - - - -   aging factors are the effect of outside influences on the skin's health.

riicnntsi

- - - - - - - - - - - - - - - - - -   aging is the part of the aging process that is due to the actual passing of the years, wearing out of the body, and hereditary factors.

lrpioaer riwnnligk

- - - - - - - - - - - - - - - - - -   lines around the mouth (often called smoker's lines, although they can occur in nonsmokers).

seastlosi

- - - - - - - - - - - - - - - - - -   means "loss of elasticity of the skin."

soitps

- - - - - - - - - - - - - - - - - -   refers to more specific areas of drooping skin, such as eyelid ptosis or breast ptosis.

yethndraoid

- - - - - - - - - - - - - - - - - -   is the decreasing ability of the skin to hold water.

lsoavdtosria

- - - - - - - - - - - - - - - - - -   dilate the blood vessels, making more blood flow through the arterial system.

cnrmiocurter

- - - - - - - - - - - - - - - - - -   is a low-level current application used to stimulate and improve the elasticity of aging and sun-damaged skin.

Word Puzzle

See if you can find terms related to skin aging in the following word search. (*Hint*: the terms are also used in the word scramble above.)

```
A  R  Y  A  M  S  B  C  M  F  K  P  F  Y  Z  D  G
N  H  B  Q  D  Q  G  A  U  L  N  E  D  U  A  G  L
C  V  A  S  O  D  I  L  A  T  O  R  S  U  R  R  Y
R  G  U  E  W  O  G  H  Y  K  C  I  E  M  O  Q  H
S  X  F  H  H  E  M  A  N  Y  U  O  Z  R  T  B  O
Y  K  L  M  A  Z  D  E  H  Y  D  R  A  T  I  O  N
L  D  A  Z  L  I  K  L  A  G  W  A  G  T  N  O  L
J  I  K  W  S  E  F  H  Y  L  T  L  S  T  E  G  I
M  Q  G  A  U  L  P  A  N  F  A     A  F  O  G  N
Q  K  A  Q  A  A  A  Q  E  K  Z  W  G  K  R  B  E
Y  A  E  O  Q  S  L  M  X  S  E  R  X  A  M  D  S
N  E  Z  T  B  T  K  Y  T  O  S  I  T  P  P  U  S
M  M  I  C  R  O  C  U  R  R  E  N  T  H  W  D  Q
R  C  I  N  O  S  S  B  I  M  D  K  N  I  N  E  B
A  P  T  O  S  I  S  G  N  A  F  L  S  E  R  O  B
C  Y  G  O  G  S  L  T  S  G  L  I  A  C  W  M  Z
R  I  R  R  B  E  N  T  I  N  I  N  L  S  E  A  A
I  N  T  R  I  N  S  I  C  D  A  G  N  H  E  M  A
```

CHAPTER 19

Sun and Sun Damage

Multiple Choice

Circle the correct answer.

1. The sun projects three kinds of rays that are considered
   A. UVB long rays. B. UVC short rays. C. UVA harmful rays. D. ultraviolet rays.

2. Pigment-producing cells located in the basal layer and upper dermis are called
   A. melanin. B. melanocytes. C. melaninites. D. hyperpigmentation.

3. A dark splotching and one of the first visible signs associated with aging is called
   A. a mole. B. a nevi. C. hyperpigmentation. D. liver spots.

4. Chloasma is caused by
   A. cumulative sun exposure. B. a bad sunburn. C. hormones. D. liver ailments.

5. Hydroquinone is
   A. an exfoliant. B. a melanin suppressant. C. a type of peel. D. a melanin-producing agent.

6. To avoid having hyperpigmentation resurface after fading we must
   A. continue using exfoliant. B. continue using the melanin suppressant.
   C. minimize sun exposure and use sunscreen. D. continue to use chemical peels.

7. Tinea versicolor is
   A. dark spots on arms and legs. B. light and dark spots on arms and legs.
   C. a fungus that creates white splotches that usually appear on the chest and back of sunbathers. D. a bacterial infection requiring a visit to a dermatologist.

8. Most sun damage
   A. occurs before the age of 18 years. B. occurs in adults during the aging process because the skin is more vulnerable.
   C. is caused by sun tanning. D. occurs as an intrinsic aging factor.

9. Dermatoheliosis is the medical term for
   A. short-term damage to the skin caused by sun exposure. B. long-term damage to the skin caused by sun exposure.
   C. skin cancer. D. skin lesions.

10. Cross-linking is associated with
    A. well-hydrated, healthy skin. B. collagen building.
    C. the use of lipid replacement. D. a process in which collagen and elastin fibrils in the dermis collapse, causing the support system for the skin to collapse.

True/False

Write T for true and F for false in the space provided.

1. ____ Basal cell carcinomas are the most common forms of skin cancer.

2. ____ Estheticians can easily tell whether a lesion is a skin cancer.

3. ____ Basal cell carcinomas are difficult to treat.

4. ____ Squamous cell carcinomas are the most deadly type of skin cancers.

5. ____ An unexplained skin bleeding or small pink or red ulcerated lesion is likely to be a squamous cell carcinoma.

6. ____ All clients with suspicious lesions should be referred to a dermatologist or qualified physician.

7. ____ A melanoma often appears as a basal cell carcinoma.

8. ____ Moh's surgery is a specialized surgical technique for removing cancerous lesions.

9. ____ Actinic keratosis is always malignant.

10. ____ Sebaceous hyperplasia is a precancerous lesion.

Short Answer

1. _____ _____ are small donut-shaped lesions that look like large open comedones surrounded by a ridge of skin.

2. Large, flat, crusty-looking brown, black-yellowish, or gray lesions that are found on the faces of older clients with sun damage are called _____ _____. They are usually harmless; however, they may turn into ____ ___ _____. Thus, they should be watched by a dermatologist.

3. _____ is a topical treatment for actinic keratosis.

4. Also known as "liver spots," ____ _____ are clumps of hyperpigmentation caused by sun damage.

5. The best hindrance to sun damage is _____.

6. _____ _____ protect against both ultraviolet A and B rays.

7. The best known physical sunscreen ingredients are ___ _____ and _____ ____. They work by _____ rays off of the skin. They are also less likely to cause _____ than the _____ _____.

8. Three ingredients that absorb and chemically neutralize the ultraviolet rays are _____ _____, and _____, also known as _____ ____.

9. SPF stands for ___ _____ ____. The number represents ___ ____ a person can stay out in the sun without _____ while using the product.

10. _____ _____ ____ means how much time passes without the skin turning red from irritation.

11. A way of classifying skin by its tendency to sunburn or tan is known as _____ ____ _____. It was developed by a dermatologist named _____ _____.

12. Self-tanning products contain _____, a chemical derived from ____ ____ or ____ that turns brown when exposed to the elements; thus when it is applied to the skin it turns a golden brown, resembling a tan.

Detail or List the Following

1. Detail the ABCDEs of melanoma.

   A. _____

   B. _____

   C. _____

   D. _____

   E. _____

2. List the Fitzpatrick Skin Types.

   A. _____

   B. _____

   C. _____

   D. _____

   E. _____

   F. _____

3. List tips for clients regarding sun exposure.

   _____

   _____

   _____

   _____

   _____

   _____

   _____

   _____

   _____

   _____

Word Scramble

Unscramble the key terms below, by using the definitions shown, and write the term inside the cells.

elanmotescy

----------------- are cells that are "pigment factories" for the skin.

elmainn

----------------- is the pigment of the skin.

hpterigmyepnaitno

----------------- refers to any condition that is characterized by more than a normal amount of melanin.

ascloamh

----------------- often called "liver spots," are dark brown patches of hyperpigmentation on the skin caused by sun overexposure.

dinqrouhoney

----------------- is a drug ingredient in melanin suppressants.

inabutr

----------------- is a melanin suppressant.

ssideirmaothloe

----------------- is the medical term describing long-term damage to the skin caused by sun exposure.

csrso-inlkgin

----------------- is a process in which collagen and elastin fibrils in the dermis collapse, causing the support system for the skin also to collapse.

elaomanm

----------------- is characterized by moles or mole-like lesions that are dark in color.

dtslasicpy

----------------- means "abnormal growth."

ersnrecacp

----------------- are conditions in cells that may become cancerous.

yrrourgsecy

----------------- is the dermatological removal of lesions by freezing, usually with liquid nitrogen.

ilflurouorca

----------------- is a topical prescription drug used to remove multiple actinic keratoses.

uestrsu

----------------- are materials used in reconnecting areas of surgical incisions.

ootncatexi

----------------- is a UVB-absorbing sunscreen ingredient.

tsocieaalt

----------------- is a UVB-absorbing sunscreen ingredient.

zoeonnbexy

----------------- is a UVB- and UVA-absorbing sunscreen ingredient.

Word Puzzle

It is important to recognize different effects of sun damage on the skin, especially skin cancers. Find terms related to sun and sun damage in the following word search. (*Hint*: the terms are also used in the word scramble above.)

```
L D A Z F L U O R O U R A C I L C Y G O G N L T
J I K W S X F H Y X L G U E M L W Y G D T D P H
M Q G A U T P A N Y A R Y A M S B C M F K F F Y
Q O A Q A R A Q Y B N H B Q D Q G A U L D N C M
O C T I N O X A T E C D F B P K A Q G A D R B G
V T Q G A S U L F N R C R Y O S U R G E R Y E M
A I K A Q A L Y A Z S H F H H E M A N Y U S Z R
A S A P A L E N E O Y L L M A Z L I U A T V D A
G A H L D N C M E N L O A Z L I K D A G W A G T
E L O R E S O R M E L A N O M A F E Y L H E M A
M A F P R U S A E S M S G A U T V R N F B H A F
L T O H Y D U C L G Q M A Q A R A M Y K E D G K
S E K O T G T R A R R A G H Y N E A U W Z G L W
I H I D H A U I N A V M Q G A I H T A G D R M K
A R H Y P E R P I G M E N T A T I O N E G Q E L
C R A S Z X E Q N M W D Q H L M Q H D Q M Q L M
H B Q P M U S M J I N E B I K Y Z E E B A O A U
T A M L E G I H G P A C R O S S - L I N K I N G
N C Y A O G N L T Y G L O G D S N I E D L I O K
Y R I S R B E N H Y D R O Q U I N O N E D U C D
M I B T M D S N L E D A Z X D Q H S M D C M Y I
M H G I P U S T U L E D A R B U T I N C U S T Q
P R E C A N C E R S D C N B O B I S W Y T V E K
E R E Q G Z C H N M R C W M Z G S B C W A R S G
```

CHAPTER 20

The New Science of Aging Skin Treatment

Multiple Choice

Circle the correct answer.

1. The inflammation cascade is
   A. a free radical.

   B. the process of sunburn and tanning of the skin.

   C. a biochemical reaction that eventually causes a breakdown of collagen and elastin fibrils.

   D. extrinsic aging.

2. Poikiloderma of Civatte is
   A. a condition in sun-damaged skin resulting in horseshoe-shaped red splotching on the neck.

   B. shiny papules on the sides of the face.

   C. redness on the sides of the face.

   D. a loss of pigment on the sides of the neck.

3. The majority of sun damage occurs
   A. while on vacation.

   B. from day-to-day exposure, such as driving to work, going to the mailbox, or taking a walk.

   C. from using tanning beds or tan-accelerating products.

   D. from UVA rays.

4. Daily exfoliation for aging skin
   A. should never be done.

   B. should be minimal.

   C. should be applied only to oily skin.

   D. improves barrier function, hydration, and intercellular lipid production.

5. With respect to aging, tretinoin has been shown to
   A. "reorganize" the skin, reestablishing a more normal epidermis, increasing blood vessel formation, increasing collagen production, and generally improving the damaged skin.

   B. cause peeling.

   C. improve skin texture but only when used with alpha hydroxy acids.

   D. "reorganize" the skin, but it is not as effective as retinol.

6. Alpha hydroxy and beta hydroxy acids are effective aging skin treatment tools for the esthetician because
   A. they help to replenish intercellular lipids that decrease with age and sun damage.

   B. they help to improve elastosis.

   C. they act as melanocyte suppressants.

   D. they are a type of vitamin A therapy.

7. If a patient is using a retinoid
   A. facial treatments must be stopped.   B. facial treatments may continue as planned.

   C. facial treatments need to be adapted by discontinuing the use of exfoliation treatments that may be too harsh on the skin.   D. facial treatments such as waxing, microdermabrasion, and peels are easily tolerated.

8. Magnesium ascorbyl phosphate, licorice extract, kojic acid, and hydroquinone are all forms of
   A. alpha hydroxy acids.   B. chemical peel ingredients.   C. keratolytics.   D. bleaching agents.

9. Microdermabrasion is
   A. a technique used to exfoliate the skin mechanically.   B. an antioxidant therapy.

   C. a technique used to peel the skin.   D. a technique used in surgery formerly known as "dermabrasion."

10. Broad-spectrum antioxidants are
    A. types of antioxidants that are used in the bleaching process.   B. types of alpha hydroxy acids.

    C. combinations of antioxidants that work together to stop the inflammation cascade of chemical reactions.   D. unstable when used on the skin.

True/False

Write T for true and F for false in the space provided.

1. ____ All antioxidants help to fight free radicals.

2. ____ Antioxidants are the same as alpha hydroxy acids.

3. ____ Liposomes provide good protection for stability of antioxidants.

4. ____ The barrier function is improved when broad-spectrum antioxidants are introduced to the skin followed by a skin condition–specific alpha hydroxy acid treatment product and broad-spectrum sunscreen.

5. ____ Powerful broad-spectrum antioxidant complexes are often manufactured in serum form.

6. ____ Peptides are used for exfoliation.

7. ____ Lipid serums for extremely dry skin are often used after sunscreen as the very last step before makeup.

8. ____ Microcurrent treatments are used to improve skin texture and elasticity.

9. ____ LED treatments are a type of laser.

10. ____ Hyperpigmentation is best treated with a comprehensive approach including chemical exfoliation, melanin suppressive agents, and sunscreens.

11. ____ Heat may cause a certain type of hyperpigmentation, even without sun exposure.

Detail, Define, or Name the Following

1. Name five basic concepts for dealing with photo-damaged skin.

   A. _____

   B. _____

   C. _____

   D. _____

   E. _____

2. Detail seven rules for working with a client using retinoids.

   A. _____

   B. _____

   _____

   C. _____

   D. _____

   _____

   E. _____

   _____

   F. _____

   _____

   _____

   G. _____

3. Define photo-damaged skin.

   _____

   _____

   _____

   _____

   _____

Word Scramble

Unscramble the key terms below, using the definitions shown, and write the term inside the cells.

zaarottnee

- - - - - - - - - - - - - - - - -

commercially known as Tazorac®, is a vitamin A-derived topical prescription medication used to treat both acne and aging symptoms caused by sun damage.

rodecrmmiasibroan

- - - - - - - - - - - - - - - - -

is a procedure using crystal particles that are pressure-sprayed onto the skin and then vacuumed. This is a mechanical exfoliation technique that removes corneum cells.

dboar-mpctersu tioxidananst

- - - - - - - - - - - - - - - - -

are a mix of various antioxidants that help neutralize or stop various free-radical reactions during the inflammation cascade.

ivanmti C

- - - - - - - - - - - - - - - - -

is a water-soluble vitamin essential in the skin for helping to neutralize free radicals; it is also needed in the production of collagen.

L-sacbocir adci

- - - - - - - - - - - - - - - - -

is a water-soluble form of vitamin C.

atviinm E

- - - - - - - - - - - - - - - - -

is a fat-soluble vitamin that is a strong antioxidant.

oocoprhtel

- - - - - - - - - - - - - - - - -

is the chemical name for vitamin E.

ptcooerlhy caeatte

- - - - - - - - - - - - - - - - -

is a more stable form of vitamin E often used in skin-care products.

chchlioalneco

- - - - - - - - - - - - - - - - -

is a powerful antioxidant derived from licorice root.

tvseraolrre

- - - - - - - - - - - - - - - - -

is a powerful antioxidant, known for its presence in red wine, but derived from plant sources for use in skin care.

idbeeeonn

- - - - - - - - - - - - - - - - -

is a powerful antioxidant.

Word Puzzle

How many terms related to the science of aging skin can you find in the following word search? (*Hint:* the terms are also used in the word scramble above.)

```
W O G B E M L W Y T G D T D P H N B M D T D
M A R R A M S B C O M F K F F Y F F H R C F
L N T O C O P H E C R O L O D U L E M D S G
K C D A B P K A Q O G A D R B G A F Y C O R
L R I F S X N M A P N B C U E M M L W Y G U
D E H H E Y U B E H S R N O Z R M A B C M S
M A R R A M S B C E M O F K F F Y F F H R C
L N M I C R O D E R M A B R A S I O N O D U
K C D A B P K A Q Y A D R E B G A F Y C O R
R L D P Z V I K L L G - A S G T T G F B P K
A E G O R I O O R A I S O V L S B A M D P N
Y P K S R T I S I C Y P D E S E A A C U H K
A D T A Z A R O T E N E A R N A E R O B I C
F N F Y R M A D F T R C D A W Y T V Q L S B
T H B A G I B L M A I T E T B I K Y C U S M
I C R D C N O A E T D R O R H W D Q H L M D
K S R U L C C M J E I U E O T A M S E G I S
D A R I M T R M M H G M P L P U S T U L E L
E I H X S H R M I B A A M D S N E E D O I Y
R S B O O T E Y R I R N R B E N N O N R T E
E L W I H Y D N C Y G T O G C L O Y G T S R
A E G N R E R O R C V I T A M I N E R I N O
N S L A M R P N A D F O E G I H G P A F O C
H G G A L D C C M E D X E E I L A R R E T A
L A D I P A Z E N E T I B M K H G O M V L A
Q V T M U G A S U L I D E B E N O N E F U R
O R O T K O T C E A R A O R T K O T C E A R
L I C H O C H A L C O N E A M R P N A D F N
Q V O E W O G U N Q V T D S E A A C U H K A
H M P R Y E W O L - A S C O R B I C A C I D
E D H S M Q C A U T P A N F A H A F I G T N
H G E Y B I Y D S E A A C U H K A Q V O R C
L M R H A Q M A Q M L Y A E O Q A L C O S S
S N O R S H R M I B A M D S N E E D O I Y D
A M L E D O H W D Q H L M D C M J S B C W A
```

CHAPTER 21

Chemical Peeling and Exfoliation Procedures

Multiple Choice

Circle the correct answer.

1. The two types of surface exfoliation are
   A. alpha hydroxy acid and beta hydroxy acid.
   B. enzyme and mechanical.
   C. chemical and mechanical.
   D. chemical and enzyme.

2. Microdermabrasion is a form of
   A. chemical exfoliation.
   B. abrasion exfoliation.
   C. mechanical exfoliation.
   D. removing dead skin cells.

3. One of the many benefits of surface exfoliation is that
   A. it thoroughly cleanses the skin.
   B. by removing the dead cell layer, the lower-level cells are moved to the surface more quickly, improving moisture content of the surface of the skin.
   C. it eliminates deeper lines.
   D. it extracts comedones more easily.

4. For a client with dry-to-normal skin, a home-care mechanical exfoliation treatment should consist of
   A. a light scrub.
   B. a peel with a pH of at least 1.5.
   C. a thicker granular scrub.
   D. a brush followed by a benzoyl peroxide cleanser.

5. Enzymes are considered
   A. a mechanical exfoliation.
   B. proteolytic.
   C. a deeper chemical peel.
   D. beta hydroxy acid.

6. Sensitive skin types can usually tolerate
   A. glycolic acid treatments.
   B. salicylic acid treatments.
   C. mechanical exfoliating treatments.
   D. enzyme treatments.

7. Usually the higher the pH in an acid peel
   A. the lower the concentration of the peel.
   B. the higher the concentration of the peel.
   C. the less irritating the peel will be.
   D. the more irritating the peel will be.

8. In salon glycolic treatments, it is important for estheticians to use a product within the range of
   A. 70 percent and 99 percent peel solution with a low pH of 2.0 or less.
   B. 8 percent and 10 percent peel solution with a high pH of 2.0 or more.
   C. 10 percent and 12 percent peel solution with a low pH of 1.0 or less.
   D. 15 percent and 30 percent solution with a high pH of 3.0 or more.

9. The three most important elements in applying glycolic acid peels are to
   A. have proper training and experience in applying them, know the type of skin you are peeling, and follow the manufacturer's recommendations.
   B. make sure that the skin you are peeling is clean and free of oil and debris, use proper pre-peel solution, and watch the timer.
   C. explain the peel procedure to the client, use the proper solution for peeling, and apply the peel solution in a uniform manner avoiding the eye area.
   D. use common sense, follow the manufacturer's recommended directions, and use a pre-peeling solution that is a keratolytic.

10. While planning an alpha hydroxy acid treatment, you notice a client has a herpetic breakout (cold sore). You should
    A. go ahead and do the treatment, avoiding the lip area.
    B. not apply the treatment, reschedule a minimum of two to three weeks ahead, and refer the client to a doctor for treatment and prophylaxis.
    C. suggest that you do a different type of treatment.
    D. follow manufacturer's instructions.

True/False

Write T for true and F for false in the space provided.

1. ____ It is important for men to avoid shaving prior to having a glycolic peel.

2. ____ Always use a sunscreen of SPF 15 or higher post-peel.

3. ____ It is not uncommon for glycolic treatments to create an increase in comedones in the beginning of a series.

4. ____ Chemical peeling may lighten hyperpigmented areas, especially if the stains are superficial.

5. ____ A phenol peel is safe enough for the esthetician to apply.

6. ____ Trichloroacetic acid peels are medium-depth peels that are performed by dermatologists and plastic surgeons.

7. ____ Laser resurfacing uses a carbon dioxide (CO_2) laser to remove layers of the epidermis.

8. ____ The removal of live tissue is in the domain of the esthetician.

9. ____ Some clients undergoing peeling treatments for acne may find it getting worse before it gets better.

10. ____ Clients with sun-damaged, hyperpigmented skin are the best candidates for superficial peeling that is offered by estheticians.

Short Answer

1. Clients who are pregnant or lactating _____ have chemical peeling.

2. Make certain that your client has begun a _____ ____ consisting of ____ _____ ____ or ___ _____ ____ _____, and _____ prior to starting chemical peeling treatments.

3. It is important to tell the client what the peel will do in a pre-peel consultation, and ____ _ ___ __ _.

4. _____ describes a white appearance of the skin that appears after applying a strong exfoliation or peeling substance.

5. If a client has a reaction to a peel, _____ refer them to a dermatologist.

6. Many estheticians are _____ at performing chemical peels. It is vitally important to train and retrain with a _____ _____.

Define, Detail, or Describe the Following

1. Define superficial peeling.

   _____

   _____

   _____

   _____

   _____

2. Define medium-depth peels.

   _____

   _____

   _____

   _____

   _____

   _____

3. Detail the benefits of surface exfoliation.

   _____

   _____

   _____

   _____

   _____

   _____

4. Detail the precautions to take when administering glycolic peelings.

   _____

   _____

   _____

   _____

   _____

   _____

   _____

   _____

5. Describe what a superficial peeling will not do.

_____

_____

_____

_____

_____

Word Scramble

Unscramble the key terms below by using the definitions shown, and write the term inside the cells.

cmhaenialc ltieoaioxfn

- - - - - - - - - - - - - - - - - -   describes any process that removes dead cells from the skin surface by physical means, such as brushing, a granular scrub, or microdermabrasion.

roicdbermmanasior

- - - - - - - - - - - - - - - - - -   is a procedure using crystal particles that are pressure-sprayed onto the skin and then vacuumed. This is a mechanical exfoliation technique that removes corneum cells.

ogmgema

- - - - - - - - - - - - - - - - - -   is a mechanical exfoliation procedure in which a paraffin-based cream is applied to the skin, allowed to dry, and then "rolled" off the skin surface, removing dead surface cells.

rgsialcu ohnple epnlieg

- - - - - - - - - - - - - - - - - -   is a very deep-peeling procedure performed by a plastic surgeon or dermatologist. The peel affects the dermis and has considerable risks.

craonb dxiidoe alser

- - - - - - - - - - - - - - - - - -   is a surgical laser used in resurfacing. It removes epidermal and dermal tissue to treat wrinkles in sun-damaged skin.

tlaeadb

- - - - - - - - - - - - - - - - - -   is a medical term meaning "removed." Tissue ablated during laser resurfacing is removed by the laser.

iavalteb

- - - - - - - - - - - - - - - - - -   is a term describing a laser that removes tissue.

muiedm-dpeht eplse

- - - - - - - - - - - - - - - - - -   are performed by dermatologists or plastic surgeons. These trichloroacetic acid (TCA) peels affect the dermis, but not as deeply as phenol.

usferipclia lpieneg

- - - - - - - - - - - - - - - - - -   affects the epidermis and is performed by estheticians or physicians. These peels include alpha and beta hydroxy acids, Jessner's solution, and resorcinol peeling treatments.

gnostrif

- - - - - - - - - - - - - - - - - -   describes a white appearance of the skin that appears after applying a strong exfoliation or peeling substance. It is caused by denaturing keratin protein in the corneum cells.

Word Puzzle

See if you can find terms related to chemical peeling and exfoliation in the following word search. (*Hint:* the terms are also used in the word scramble above.)

```
T  M D  M E  D I  U M - D E P  T H P E  E L S  A E R K K U D
M Y C E O S R I  U M A R S  M F L I  H B Q G A G R S Q G
U  W Y C U U O U D E Q A C H U H K N D F B A E N I  M U
U  O C H S  S C S C E K M A Z U L M T G E Q G L D T I  R
E  N T A R O A N X H Y P E G R K E I  A T O S I  S T C I
B  T F N B Y R G H T C F R O S T I  N G Q A R A O U R S
L  C G I  H H B O S H Y B K M C M H K C S D I  S M C O L
M Y C C O S O I  U M A R S  M F L I  H B Q G A G R S D G
U  W Y A U U N U D E A B L A T I  V E D F B A E N I  E U
E  N T L R O D N X H B P E G R K E I  A T O S I  S T R I
S  U P E R F I  C I  A L P E E L I  N G F L I  H B Q G M A
B  T F X B Y O G H T A K E I  A T O S T Q A R A O U A S
U  O C F S  S X S C E T M A Z U L M T G E Q G L D T B R
M Y C O O S I  I  U M E R S  M F L I  H B Q G A G R S R G
L  C G L H H D O S H D B K U C M H K C S D I  S M C A L
T  M D I  R O E M A Z U L M T G I  H B R U A E R K K S D
U  W Y A U U L U D E Q A C H U H K N D F B A E N I  I  U
M Y C T O S A I  U M A R S  M F L I  H B Q G A G R S O G
E  N T I  R O S U R G I  C A L P H E N O L P E E L I  N G
B  T F O B Y E G H T C S  M F L I  H B R Q A R A O U Q S
M Y C N O S R I  U M A R S  M F L I  H B Q G A G R S Q G
```

CHAPTER 22

Plastic and Cosmetic Surgery: Treating the Patient

Multiple Choice

Circle the correct answer.

1. To the postoperative patient, the esthetician can play a significant role
   A. as health educator and as psychological support.
   B. as support to the physician by taking out sutures and staples.
   C. as the key point person in all postoperative visits.
   D. as health educator and counselor or advisor.

2. The two types of cosmetic surgery are
   A. cosmetic and plastic.
   B. cosmetic and reconstructive.
   C. reconstructive and endoscopic.
   D. cosmetic and rejuvenating.

3. Cosmetic surgery generally refers to
   A. skin cancer removal.
   B. surgical procedures that correct abnormalities.
   C. surgical procedures used for cosmetic purposes.
   D. reconstructive surgery.

4. Reconstructive surgery refers to
   A. primarily cosmetic surgery.
   B. primarily skin cancer.
   C. face lifts and eye lifts.
   D. surgical procedure techniques used to correct noncosmetic abnormalities, such as skin cancer removal, or surgery needed as a result of accidental injury or other physical deformities.

5. A general plastic surgeon
   A. performs primarily facial plastic surgery.
   B. performs primarily eyelid surgery.
   C. performs all types of plastic, reconstructive, and cosmetic surgery.
   D. performs primarily face lifts.

6. Sutures are
   A. materials used in reconnecting areas of surgical incisions.
   B. materials used in providing relief from swelling or edema.
   C. materials used in face lift surgery.
   D. mostly dissolvable.

7. A midface lift is
   A. a newer procedure that involves primarily the contour of the area just under the cheekbone and lifting the nasolabial folds.
   B. a newer procedure that affects primarily the jaw line and neck regions.
   C. a newer procedure that affects the nasal region.
   D. a procedure that requires less downtime and creates less bruising and swelling.

8. Immediate postoperative care will be delivered by
   A. the esthetician.   B. the nurse.   C. the anesthesiologist.   D. the physician.

9. Long-term skin-care needs for the surgical patient are
   A. minimal and not really necessary.
   B. important to protect the appearance and investment in the surgery.
   C. important to hide the scars from the surgery.
   D. minimal but new hairstyles become important.

10. The surgical procedure for lifting the eye and removing excess skin from the eye area is called
    A. a rhytidectomy.   B. a rhinoplasty.   C. a blepharoplasty.   D. an endoscopic procedure.

True/False

Write T for true and F for false in the space provided.

1. ____ A blepharoplasty will correct puffy, baggy, and droopy eyelids.

2. ____ A forehead lift helps to correct elastosis of the eyebrows.

3. ____ Most numbing created by surgical procedures subsides over time.

4. ____ The surgical term used for a "nose job" is rhytidectomy.

5. ____ The "thread lift" is a less invasive procedure for lifting the skin of the cheeks and jaw line.

6. ____ Microdermabrasion is a technique of reducing acne scarring, scar tissue, and deep wrinkles.

7. ____ Laser resurfacing is a technique used to retexturize the surface of the skin and "plane down" wrinkles.

8. ____ Glycolic peels are an excellent preoperative treatment for laser resurfacing.

9. ____ Microdermabrasion, light peels, or brushing can be used immediately post-laser resurfacing.

10. ____ Hyperpigmentation may be created by laser resurfacing, and hydroquinone may be used to lighten the areas along with daily sunscreen use.

Fill in the Blank

Using the word bank below, fill in the blank to complete the sentence. The same word or phrase may be used more than once.

Word Bank

treatment methods	swelling	intradermal	facial expressions	skin-care instruction
milia	frowning	rhytidectomy	contraindicated	treatments
liposuction	Botox®	implants	returning	lifestyle
recovering	deposits	manual lymphatic	hyaluronic acid	side effects
quickly	paralysis	drainage	sun protection	
daily	esthetician			

1. Many in-office _____ _____ may be used to help minimize redness and _____ after surgical procedures. It will be important to follow the attending physician's requirements postsurgically because some _____ may be _____ while the client is _____ from a procedure.

2. _____ _____ _____ is an excellent treatment, following a face lift or _____, to reduce swelling and stiffness.

3. One of the most important skin treatment products to use postsurgically is ___ _____. It must be used ____ following the surgeon's protocol.

4. The _____ is of great help to the patient and the physician by removing _____, which can easily form during the healing phase after a laser resurfacing procedure. In addition, _____ _____ and direction can be provided by the _____, which many physicians support and for which they are grateful.

5. _____ is the term for surgical removal of fat _____.

6. The term _____ refers to inside the dermis and is often associated with filler material that may be injected to fill in wrinkles, scars, and depressions.

7. Small sacks of silicone or saline that are placed in the cheek, chin, and breasts are called _____.

8. _____ _____ is a popular injectable being used as a filler with little to no ____ _____.

9. Botulinum toxin is commonly known as _____. It causes a temporary _____ of the muscle, thus preventing certain ____ _____ such as _____.

10. One of the most important factors to the patient following a surgical procedure is _____ to a normal _____ as _____ as possible.

Define, Detail, or Name the Following

1. Detail a home-care plan for the patient post-laser surgery.

_____

_____

_____

_____

_____

_____

2. Define cosmetic surgery.

_____

_____

_____

_____

_____

3. Define reconstructive surgery.

_____

_____

_____

_____

_____

_____

4. Name the common types of cosmetic surgery.

_____

_____

_____

_____

_____

_____

_____

_____

Word Scramble

Unscramble the key terms below by using the definitions shown, and write the terms inside the cells.

myyrheidctto

- - - - - - - - - - - - - - - - - is the medical term for a face lift.

dmi-acef flit

- - - - - - - - - - - - - - - - - is a surgical procedure used to lift the middle section of the face.

nicaar mtaonan

- - - - - - - - - - - - - - - - - is a homeopathic herb also used to control and speed healing.

amukep onter

- - - - - - - - - - - - - - - - - is a colored liquid or cream foundation that is used to neutralize unnatural skin colors such as bruising or redness.

yephabloaplsrt

- - - - - - - - - - - - - - - - - is the surgical procedure for "lifting" the eyes and removing excess skin from the eye area.

efohedra ftil

- - - - - - - - - - - - - - - - - is a surgical procedure that helps correct elastosis of the forehead and lift the brows.

htreda ilitngf

- - - - - - - - - - - - - - - - - is a less invasive procedure for lifting the skin of the cheeks and jaw line.

aremrasbiodn

- - - - - - - - - - - - - - - - - is the technique of reducing acne scarring; scar tissue; and, in some cases, wrinkles.

labtiaev alers

- - - - - - - - - - - - - - - - - removes or "evaporates" skin cells. In laser resurfacing, the laser is used to retexturize the surface of the skin, literally vaporizing layers of skin.

rcftinaola aslre

- - - - - - - - - - - - - - - - - sometimes called by its trademark name Fraxel®, are used to treat wrinkles, photo damage, mild scarring, and hyperpigmentation. This laser is split into thousands of columns. The method provides results over a series of treatments with less severe and fewer side effects and downtime.

politiosucn

- - - - - - - - - - - - - - - - - is the term for surgical removal of fat deposits.

tsmaplni

- - - - - - - - - - - - - - - - - are small silicone or saline "sacks" used to improve the appearance of the cheeks and chin.

lliersf

- - - - - - - - - - - - - - - - - are materials used to fill wrinkles and skin depressions by injection or implantation.

ritamderlna

- - - - - - - - - - - - - - - - - means "inside the dermis," which is where collagen and other filler material may be injected to fill out hypotrophic scars, wrinkles, or pock marks.

clolaeng tijnecinso

- - - - - - - - - - - - - - - - - are procedures performed by a plastic surgeon; they involve injecting collagen into depression scars or wrinkles to reduce the appearance of the lesion.

tfa tnecijonis

- - - - - - - - - - - - - - - - - are filling injections using the patient's own fat to fill depressions and wrinkles.

tbulioumn ioxnt

- - - - - - - - - - - - - - - - - is the toxin used in Botox.

lagelbal

- - - - - - - - - - - - - - - - - is the muscle between the eyes that frequently causes expression lines in the forehead area. This area is frequently treated with Botox®.

Word Puzzle

See if you can find cosmetic surgery related terms in the following word search. (*Hint*: the terms are also used in the word scramble above.)

```
C O S R I U M A R S M F L G H B Q G A R I H B Q G M G R
E C I T A R G O M M A G E L P I A I K U O P K A I I K D
T R O A F A T I N J E C T I O N S I S C I A T S I D T E
G O H L M O S M Y B G C M P K T D I S C H K C D I - M R
S D Y A G C R P X L A T E O K R A O G C M A B Y A F C M
E C I T A R G L M M A G E S P A R N I C A M O N T A N A
C O S R C U M A R S M F L U H D Q G A R K H T Q G C G B
R F I C O A L N P E E L I C G E A A T L E D U H L E D R
G O H L L O S T Y B G C M T K R D F S C U K L D I L M A
T R O A L I S S C I A B S I T M T O I C P H I Q I I T S
Q H L M A C U J I K P L X O H A Y R G A T A N S I F C I
T E S I G C R U S T A E I N N L A E R I O O U X A T L O
H R F I E I A L G P E P L I N G T H A T N I M H I L M N
R C I A N H L M L K P H Y B G C M E I C E A T Y B G C M
E T R O I Q H L A B L A T I V E L A S E R T O N G T H I
A R F I N C U J B P E R C R U S T D Y B G C X C R U S T
D P E E J B G C E K P O Y B F I L L E R S C I L I N G T
L S T A E O H L L C R P M M A G E I A A T L N Q G A R U
I Q H L C R F I L C U L X L A T E F Q G A R I H B Q G Q
F R A C T I O N A L L A S E R L M T Y B G C M I N G T R
T H L M I C Y B G C M S S R I U M A R S M F L G H G C M
I P E E O C U J R H Y T I D E C T O M Y D I S C H K C D
N C O S N C U J I K P Y Y B G C M M A R S M F L G H G C
G G O H S M O S L R G O M M A G E S R I U M A R D I S H
```

CHAPTER 23

Cosmetic Medicine and Medical Relations

Multiple Choice

Circle the correct answer.

1. Cosmetic dermatology is a
   A. subspecialty of plastic surgery.
   B. subspecialty of otolaryngology.
   C. subspecialty of dermatology.
   D. form of Moh's surgery.

2. Internists specialize in
   A. diseases such as rheumatoid arthritis and lupus.
   B. internal diseases such as heart problems, diabetes, and other internal afflictions.
   C. the treatment of the endocrine system.
   D. the treatment of advanced skin disease.

3. Estheticians are licensed to provide
   A. all services that are offered in the practice.
   B. noninvasive, topical services and those that are supervised by a physician.
   C. noninvasive, topical services that are within the scope of the licensed esthetician, as defined by the state board of cosmetology.
   D. treatments that involve only the epidermis and dermis.

4. Estheticians may be allowed to operate lasers
   A. if the state in which they are practicing allows it.
   B. if the state in which they are practicing allows it, they have been certified to do so, and they are under the supervision of a qualified medical physician.
   C. if they have been certified according to manufacturer's specifications.
   D. if they have been certified by a physician.

5. Nonablative lasers
   A. do not destroy tissue or peel the skin to any degree.
   B. are lasers used to vaporize the skin.
   C. are strictly for exfoliation.
   D. are for use in laser resurfacing.

6. Intense pulsed light is
   A. a type of laser that is used for hyperpigmentation and telangiectasias.
   B. a type of light therapy that is used for hyperpigmentation and telangiectasias.
   C. a radio frequency heat treatment that is used to stimulate collagen.
   D. used for skin tags and moles.

7. Thermage® is a trademarked name for a medical procedure used to stimulate collagen with
   A. light waves.
   B. a specified laser.
   C. an Nd:YAG.
   D. radio frequency.

True/False

Write T for true and F for false in the space provided.

1. ____ Estheticians who are certified in medical procedures such as laser hair removal are allowed to practice them if the state in which they are practicing allows it and they are working under the supervision of a qualified medical physician.

2. ____ If the state in which an esthetician is licensed does not allow for an esthetician to use laser therapy, it is legal if it is done in a medical office under the supervision of a qualified medical physician.

3. ____ To date, there is no state that recognizes the title "paramedical esthetician."

4. ____ Services that involve treatments below the surface of the skin or on live tissue are considered invasive and are not to be administered by estheticians.

5. ____ Availability is one of the key reasons that dermatologists recommend soap and water to their patients for cleansing.

Define, Name, or Detail the Following

1. Define cosmetic dermatology.

_____

_____

_____

_____

2. Define "scope of practice."

_____

_____

_____

_____

3. Name what the letters in laser stand for.

_____

_____

_____

_____

4. Detail briefly how a laser works.

_____

_____

_____

_____

5. Detail briefly the steps to referring a client to a physician.

_____

_____

_____

_____

_____

_____

_____

_____

Word Scramble

Unscramble the key terms below using the definitions shown, and write the terms inside the cells.

omsh' gsresoun

- - - - - - - - - - - - - - - - - -   are dermatologists specially trained in a precise form of surgery to remove skin cancers.

giocrdiennolosst

- - - - - - - - - - - - - - - - - -   specialize in treating diseases of the endocrine system.

umrhestsatogilo

- - - - - - - - - - - - - - - - - -   are specialists in rheumatoid diseases, including lupus.

stenistrin

- - - - - - - - - - - - - - - - - -   specialize in treating internal diseases, including heart problems, diabetes, and other internal afflictions.

snnvaivenio

- - - - - - - - - - - - - - - - - -   describes procedures that do not break the skin.

cosep fo trpcicae

- - - - - - - - - - - - - - - - - -   describes services allowed to be performed under a specific license.

snaiivev

- - - - - - - - - - - - - - - - - -   describes procedures that break the skin.

etcosicm gadrmeoloty

- - - - - - - - - - - - - - - - - -   is a subspecialty of dermatology treating appearance-oriented problems of the skin.

emaicld saps

- - - - - - - - - - - - - - - - - -   are medical offices that offer medical esthetic procedures beyond the scope of routine esthetic services.

nanaoltbiev

- - - - - - - - - - - - - - - - - -   describes a procedure that does not remove tissue.

bataivel

- - - - - - - - - - - - - - - - - -   is a term describing a laser that removes tissue.

toerhcen

- - - - - - - - - - - - - - - - - -   describes extremely concentrated light.

plderaganinm

- - - - - - - - - - - - - - - - - -   is a procedure that involves carefully planing the facial skin with a scalpel-like instrument before using alpha or beta hydroxy acid peels.

oetecrl-toipcla yrsnegy

- - - - - - - - - - - - - - - - - -   is a medical technique of treating cosmetic disorders using a combination of light and radio frequency energy.

Word Puzzle

See if you can find terms related to cosmetic medicine and medical relations in the following word search. (*Hint:* the terms are also used in the word scramble above.)

```
R O G H Y N P E L E C T R O - O P T I C A L S Y N E R G Y
A Q K A Q A L Y A E O Q H L M O S E N O B C U L E M D S G
G G H L D N C M E D E E I L E R O I V R A N M M L W Y G U
R A N M M L O R C I L O L S L A N D A N N W Y G U O B C U
E G O R E S R H E U M A T O L O G I S T S L R M A B C M S
R O G H S N P H W K O M N G M N C Y I M N G M N B M D T D
U W A G C R E L C O H E R E N T B M V A E O Q H L M O S E
O R C I O L N R C I S O N N D G G H E D N C M E D E E I L
G G H L P N D M E D S E O O E R O A E G O R E S O R C I R
D C E G E S O R C I U O N E R N B B R O E D E E I L E R O
R E S O O L C R O G R C I O M E G L G I I H U W A G L W K
R O G H F N R H P R G F N E A Y C A M N N G M N B M D T D
U J I K P W I S X F E H V L P E G T Y T S E A A C U H K A
X Y K L R M N A Z N O N A B L A T I V E R O B I C W Y T V
L I U A A V O R N A N Q S E A T Y V A R G G H L D N C M E
M E D I C A L S P A S D I A N Q K E A N Q A L Y A E O Y A
L W O G T D O T D P H E V M I T C T C I N O P S B A M D P
B D I K I R G A D R B G E F N C O D I S R R B C N T O N I
A G A Y C T I E Z L T U A T G D A A C T E A N L O H W V N
K A R G E D S B G A F Y C O A D I R R S B C N T O N I T E
E G O R E S T R C I O O L S L A N D E G O R E S O R C I R
B G A R C O S M E T I C D E R M A T O L O G Y T D P H E G
```

CHAPTER 24

The Scientific Approach

Multiple Choice

Circle the correct answer.

1. An essential part of professional growth is
   A. improving your sales techniques.
   B. improving your education.
   C. sharing with others.
   D. finding new clients.

2. The scientific method refers to
   A. variables in an experiment.
   B. the experimental technique that proves precise measurements.
   C. the experimental technique of developing a hypothesis or ideas, based on available information.
   D. a hypothesis in an experiment.

3. A control group is
   A. a group that changes behavior in a study.
   B. a group that is carefully selected to participate in a study.
   C. a group that is not characteristic of other groups in the study.
   D. a group in an experiment that does not change behavior.

4. A placebo is
   A. a fake product or substance used in a study.
   B. a true product or substance used in a study.
   C. a by-product of a substance used in a study.
   D. a calculation of a product or substance used in a study.

5. Puffing is a term used to describe
   A. filling a product with a substance that it is missing.
   B. making a product sound much better than it truly is.
   C. making a product pass certain tests in scientific studies.
   D. competitors making a product sound worse than it is.

6. Anecdotal evidence is
   A. evidence that is based on observation and theory but has not been thoroughly tested scientifically.
   B. evidence that has been thoroughly examined scientifically.
   C. evidence that has been used in the making of pharmaceuticals.
   D. information that has been used in the making of natural products.

True/False

Write T for true and F for false in the space provided.

1. ____ An example of anecdotal evidence would be that the skin of many of your clients with acne clears up with the use of a specific cleanser that you are using in your practice.

2. ____ If there is a measurable difference in factors before and after an experiment, the results are said to be statistically significant.

3. ____ Advertisements for products making claims like a "skin cream miracle" or a "face lift in a jar" are examples of puffing.

4. ____ Natural cosmetics are superior products to those made with chemicals.

5. ____ If a company makes a claim that a product has an effect on the functioning of the body, it is making drug claims.

6. ____ Basic skin-care training offers enough hours of specialized instruction necessary to practice advanced clinical skin care.

7. ____ One of the biggest functions of professional organizations is that they serve as legislative "watchdogs" for the profession.

8. ____ EstheticsAmerica is the esthetics division of the National Cosmetology Association (NCA).

Describe, Detail, or Name the Following

1. Describe the scientific method.

   _____

   _____

   _____

   _____

2. Detail the difference between scientific and anecdotal evidence.

   _____

   _____

   _____

   _____

3. Name the three special secrets to being a successful esthetician.

   A. _____

   B. _____

   C. _____

   _____

Word Scramble

Unscramble the key terms below using the definitions shown, and write the terms inside the cells.

tificenisc htodem

- - - - - - - - - - - - - - - - - refers to the experimental technique of developing a hypothesis, or idea, based on available information. The hypothesis is tested and interpreted, and results are published.

torlnoc ouprg

- - - - - - - - - - - - - - - - - is the group in an experiment that has no change in its behavior during the experiment.

aceoblp

- - - - - - - - - - - - - - - - - describes a substance used in an experiment that does not contain the ingredient thought to achieve a change.

tiscitstas

- - - - - - - - - - - - - - - - - are precise mathematical measurements of changes in an experiment.

ffginup

- - - - - - - - - - - - - - - - - is a term used to describe the way some companies make their products sound better than they are.

Word Puzzle

Identify the terms related to the scientific method in the following word search. (*Hint*: the terms are also used in the word scramble above.)

```
S  A  L  V  G  N  E  S  K  K  C  R  E  A  M  S
T  B  R  E  A  G  T  I  P  L  A  C  E  B  O  R
A  P  G  O  T  R  G  C  U  P  E  D  D  X  B  H
T  F  R  W  C  V  E  W  F  H  E  S  D  L  G  J
I  W  M  E  O  C  Q  O  F  Q  F  M  B  G  S  N
S  C  I  E  N  T  I  F  I  C  M  E  T  H  O  D
T  D  G  F  T  Q  A  I  N  C  C  R  A  H  M  S
I  K  F  T  R  A  D  C  G  A  X  V  S  G  M  E
C  L  V  P  O  G  Q  M  L  S  E  R  U  M  S  D
S  M  Q  C  L  A  Q  H  M  P  O  U  L  E  D  B
F  R  W  V  G  W  N  H  E  S  D  L  G  J  Z  J
F  R  W  V  R  W  N  H  E  S  D  L  G  J  Z  J
Z  E  M  Q  O  R  Q  Q  D  M  P  O  N  L  E  S
V  G  G  B  U  E  M  E  F  B  E  H  K  S  K  S
R  V  D  D  P  P  R  L  K  O  H  P  L  E  B  Q
```

CPSIA information can be obtained
at www.ICGtesting.com
Printed in the USA
FFOW03n0438260314
4527FF